Manual of Essential
Hypertension

Manual of Essential Hypertension

Nihar Mehta MD DNB (Medicine)
DNB (Cardiology) FRCP (London) FICP
Consultant Interventional Cardiologist and
Structural Heart Disease Specialist,
Jaslok, Breach Candy, HN Reliance,
Bhatia, St Elizabeth and
KJ Somaiya Superspecialty Hospitals
Mumbai, Maharashtra, India

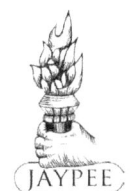

JAYPEE BROTHERS MEDICAL PUBLISHERS
The Health Sciences Publisher
New Delhi | London

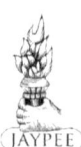 **Jaypee Brothers Medical Publishers (P) Ltd**

Headquarters
EMCA House
23/23-B, Ansari Road, Daryaganj
New Delhi 110 002, India
Landline: +91-11-23272143, +91-11-23272703
+91-11-23282021, +91-11-23245672
E-mail: jaypee@jaypeebrothers.com

Corporate Office
Jaypee Brothers Medical Publishers (P) Ltd.
4838/24, Ansari Road, Daryaganj
New Delhi 110 002, India
Phone: +91-11-43574357
Fax: +91-11-43574314
E-mail: jaypee@jaypeebrothers.com

Overseas Office
JP Medical Ltd.
83, Victoria Street, London
SW1H 0HW (UK)
Phone: +44-20 3170 8910
Fax: +44(0)20 3008 6180
E-mail: info@jpmedpub.com

Website: www.jaypeebrothers.com
Website: www.jaypeedigital.com

© 2023, Jaypee Brothers Medical Publishers

The views and opinions expressed in this book are solely those of the original contributor(s)/author(s) and do not necessarily represent those of editor(s) or publisher of the book.

All rights reserved by the author. No part of this publication may be reproduced, stored or transmitted in any form or by any means, electronic, mechanical, photocopying, recording or otherwise, without the prior permission in writing of the publishers.

All brand names and product names used in this book are trade names, service marks, trademarks or registered trademarks of their respective owners. The publisher is not associated with any product or vendor mentioned in this book.

Medical knowledge and practice change constantly. This book is designed to provide accurate, authoritative information about the subject matter in question. However, readers are advised to check the most current information available on procedures included and check information from the manufacturer of each product to be administered, to verify the recommended dose, formula, method and duration of administration, adverse effects and contraindications. It is the responsibility of the practitioner to take all appropriate safety precautions. Neither the publisher nor the author(s)/editor(s) assume any liability for any injury and/or damage to persons or property arising from or related to use of material in this book.

This book is sold on the understanding that the publisher is not engaged in providing professional medical services. If such advice or services are required, the services of a competent medical professional should be sought.

Every effort has been made where necessary to contact holders of copyright to obtain permission to reproduce copyright material. If any have been inadvertently overlooked, the publisher will be pleased to make the necessary arrangements at the first opportunity.

Inquiries for bulk sales may be solicited at: jaypee@jaypeebrothers.com

Manual of Essential Hypertension / Nihar Mehta

First Edition: 2023

ISBN: 978-93-89587-38-8

Dedicated to

All past, present and future patients suffering from hypertension
Hoping for better management and control

Contributors

Amit A Saraf MD FRCP (London, Edinburgh, Glasgow) FACP (Philadelphia) FICP FCPS
Director
Department of Internal Medicine
Jupiter Hospital
Mumbai, Maharashtra, India

Amjad Khan DNB (Nephrology)
Nephrologist and Transplant Physician
Department of Nephrology
Jaslok Hospital and Research Centre
Mumbai, Maharashtra, India

Anand Bhabhor MD IDCCM
Additional Director and Consultant
Critical Care Medicine
Jaslok Hospital and Research Centre
Mumbai, Maharashtra, India

Mitul A Shah DNB (Cardiology) DNB (Medicine)
Consultant Cardiologist
Department of Cardiology
Fortis Hospital
Mumbai, Maharashtra, India

Nandhakumar Vasu MD DNB (Cardiology) FNB (Interventional Cardiology)
Consultant Cardiologist
Department of Cardiology
Institute of Cardio Vascular Diseases
Madras Medical Mission
Chennai, Tamil Nadu, India

Nihar Mehta MD DNB (Medicine) DNB (Cardiology) FRCP (London) FICP
Consultant Interventional Cardiologist and Structural Heart Disease Specialist
Jaslok, Breach Candy, HN Reliance Bhatia, St Elizabeth and KJ Somaiya Superspecialty Hospitals
Mumbai, Maharashtra, India

Nikesh Jain DNB (Medicine) DNB (Cardiology)
Consultant Cardiologist
Department of Cardiology
Jaslok Hospital and Research Centre
Mumbai, Maharashtra, India

Nimish Shah MBBS MRCP (UK) MRCP (Respiratory) PG Certificate in Clinical Education
Consultant in Pulmonary and Sleep Medicine, Respiratory Medicine
Jaslok Hospital and Research Centre
Sir HN Reliance Foundation Hospital
Mumbai, Maharashtra, India

Ruchit Shah MBBS DNB (Medicine) DNB (Cardiology) FESC
Fellowship in Interventions (South Korea), Fellowship in Structural Heart Diseases (TAVR, MitraClip) LA, USA
Structural and Interventional Cardiologist
Structural and Interventional Cardiology
Saifee, Jaslok, Breach Candy, Wockhardt, Masina
Mumbai, Maharashtra, India

Shivani Kamat MD (Anesthesia)
Fellowship in Liver Transplant and
Critical Care (Medanta – The Medicity, Gurugram)
Fellowship in Liver Transplant and
Obstetric Anesthesia
(Queen Elizabeth Hospital, Birmingham Women's Hospital, UK)
Consultant
Department of Anesthesia and
Pain management, Sir HN Reliance Foundation Hospital
Mumbai, Maharashtra, India

Srinivasan Narayanan MD DNB
FNB (Interventional Cardiology)
Senior Consultant
Madras Medical Mission
Chennai, Tamil Nadu, India

Sudhiranjan Dash Choudhury
MBBS MD (Medicine) DNB (Nephrology) MNAMS
Senior Consultant and HOD
Department of Nephrology
Jaslok Hospital and Research Center
Mumbai, Maharashtra, India

Vibhor Pardasani DM (Neurology)
Consultant and Assistant Professor
Department of Neurology
Bombay Hospital Institute of Medical Sciences
Mumbai, Maharashtra, India

Zakiya E Patni BHMS
Clinical Assistant
Peddar Road Superspecialty Clinic
Mumbai, Maharashtra, India

Preface

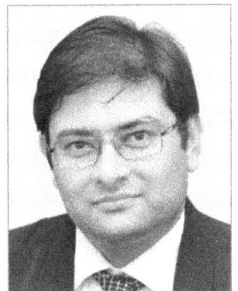

Manual of Essential Hypertension gives an in-depth understanding about high blood pressure, review of antihypertensive drugs in detail, and hypertension in various circumstances with one chapter dedicated to each special condition.

The aim is to publish a book for medical students and general physicians to help them manage hypertension effectively which even though is one of the most prevalent conditions globally and in India remains a leading cause for end organ damage due to its asymptomatic nature. Hence, in this book great emphasis has been put upon the practical aspects of diagnosis, screening, and follow-up in hypertensive management.

The management of hypertension has been emphasized through chapters on individual drugs as well as a chapter on the approach to a patient with high blood pressure. The section on special subsets gives an approach to manage high blood pressure in various clinical scenarios such as ischemic heart disease, heart failure, chronic kidney disease, respiratory disease, diabetes mellitus, obesity cerebrovascular disease, and pregnancy.

The book is written keeping in mind the medical students, hence, the MCQs and a short summary at the end of each chapter. Figures, tables, and images have been added for understanding and interpretation of various signs, symptoms, and investigations of patients and aid in their management.

Dr Amit A Saraf and Dr Ruchit Shah have contributed with chapters as well as being sectional editors. I would like to thank Dr Anand Bhabhor, Dr Nikesh Jain, Dr Amjad Khan, Dr Mitul A Shah, Dr Vibhor Pardasani, Dr Nimish Shah, Dr Shivani Kamat, Dr Sudhiranjan Dash Choudhury, Dr Srinivasan Narayanan, and Dr Nandhakumar Vasu for their valuable time and contribution to the book. Despite their busy schedules, they have given their best efforts to make this book a complete guide to daily blood pressure management. Special thanks to Dr Zakiya E Patni who has amalgamated the book by extensive proofreading in addition to the contribution to chapters.

My appreciation to the whole team of M/s Jaypee Brothers Medical Publishers (P) Ltd, New Delhi, India, for their patience, encouragement, and professionalism during the entire process. I am thankful to Shri Jitender P Vij (Group Chairman), Mr Ankit Vij (Managing Director), Mr MS Mani (Group President), Ms Chetna Malhotra (Senior Director—Professional Publishing, Marketing, and Business Development), Ms Pooja Bhandari (Production Head), and Mr Anand Kumar (Development Editor) for wonderfully framing this book within a short duration.

Special thanks goes to my family Mrs Suman Kothari, Dr Shilpa Mehta, Mrs Labdhi Mehta, Keya, Kimaya, and Raahi for their never-ending support.

Nihar Mehta

Contents

Chapter 1	**Defining and Measuring Blood Pressure** Amit A Saraf, Nikesh Jain, Nihar Mehta	1
Chapter 2	**Clinical Features and Investigations** Nikesh Jain	18
Chapter 3	**Lifestyle Management** Ruchit Shah	24
Chapter 4	**Drug Therapy** Ruchit Shah, Nihar Mehta	29
	4.1: Angiotensin-converting Enzyme Inhibitors, Angiotensin Receptor Blockers, and Renin Inhibitors Ruchit Shah	31
	4.2: Calcium Channel Blockers Ruchit Shah	38
	4.3: Diuretics Amjad Khan	42
	4.4: Beta-blockers Ruchit Shah	48
	4.5: Other Drugs Sudhiranjan Dash Choudhury, Ruchit Shah	53
	4.6: Newer Therapies for Systemic Hypertension: Renal Denervation Therapy and Baroreceptor Activation Therapy Ruchit Shah, Srinivasan Narayanan	57
Chapter 5	**Special Subsets** Amit A Saraf, Nihar Mehta	63
	5.1: Hypertension in Obesity and Metabolic Syndrome Amit A Saraf, Nimish Shah	65
	5.2: Hypertension in Special Subsets: Cerebrovascular Disease Vibhor Pardasani	70
	5.3: Hypertensive Emergency Anand Bhabhor	74

5.4:	Hypertension and Diabetes *Mitul A Shah*	80
5.5:	Hypertension and Heart Failure *Mitul A Shah*	84
5.6:	Hypertension and Pregnancy *Anand Bhabhor*	88
5.7:	Hypertension in Chronic Kidney Disease *Sudhiranjan Dash Choudhury*	94
5.8:	Perioperative Hypertension *Shivani Kamat*	101
5.9:	Hypertension in Special Subsets: Ischemic Heart Disease *Ruchit Shah, Nandhakumar Vasu*	109
5.10:	Management of Hypertension in Pulmonary Diseases *Nimish Shah*	116
5.11:	Resistant Hypertension *Amjad Khan*	121

Chapter 6   **Overview of Guidelines on Management of Hypertension**   **129**
Nihar Mehta, Zakiya E Patni

Index   **145**

CHAPTER 1

Defining and Measuring Blood Pressure

Amit A Saraf, Nikesh Jain, Nihar Mehta

INTRODUCTION

Several studies have demonstrated the association of higher systolic blood pressure (SBP) and diastolic blood pressure (DBP) with increased cardiovascular disease (CVD) risk. Increase in the SBP/DBP by 20/10 mm Hg leads to a doubling of the risk of heart diseases and strokes. Higher SBP and DBP have been associated with increased risk of angina, myocardial infarction (MI), heart failure (HF), stroke, peripheral vascular disease (PVD), and abdominal aortic aneurysm.[1,2]

WHAT IS NORMAL BLOOD PRESSURE?

Making the distinction between normal blood pressure (BP) and high BP based on a single cut-off value is quite arbitrary. Nevertheless, a cut-off value is required for simplifying the diagnosis and decision to treat high BP. Various international associations have different cut-offs based on the value above which the benefits of treatment outweigh the risks of treatment as documented by clinical trials.

Recently, the American College of Cardiology/American Heart Association (ACC/AHA) guidelines have changed the definition of normal BP to <120/80 mm Hg and the cut-off of hypertension to BP ≥130 mm Hg SBP and 90 mm Hg DBP.[1] However, the Indian Guidelines on Hypertension-IV (IGH-IV-2019)[1] and the European Society of Cardiology/European Society of Hypertension (ESC/ESH) guidelines on arterial hypertension (2018)[1] retain the earlier cut-off of ≥140/90 mm Hg for diagnosis of hypertension.

Definition

High BP in adults more than 18 years of age is defined as:
- SBP ≥140 mm Hg
- DBP ≥90 mm Hg
- Patient taking antihypertensive medications

Classification

Based on office BP, **Table 1** is used to classify BP into optimal, normal, high normal, and various stages of hypertension.

The accuracy of office BP has been increasingly questioned. Out-of-office BP measurements: Ambulatory blood pressure monitoring (ABPM) or home blood pressure monitoring (HBPM) are more representative of daily variations and use a larger number of BP values. ABPM and HBPM have different cut-offs for high BP as shown in **Table 2**.

TABLE 1: Classification of office blood pressure (BP) in adults aged 18 years and above.*[1]

Category	Systolic BP (mm Hg)	Diastolic BP (mm Hg)
Optimal	<120	<80
Normal	<130	<85
High normal	130–139	85–89
Hypertension		
Stage 1	140–159	90–99
Stage 2	160–179	100–109
Stage 3	≥180	≥110
Isolated systolic hypertension	≥140	<90

*Based on two/three office/clinic BP readings.

TABLE 2: Definition of high blood pressure (BP) as per office, ambulatory and home BP measurements.

Category	Systolic BP (mm Hg)	Diastolic BP (mm Hg)
Office BP	≥140	≥90
Ambulatory BP		
24 hours mean	≥130	≥80
Day-time mean	≥135	≥85
Night-time mean	≥120	≥70
Home BP mean	≥135	≥85

PRIMARY AND SECONDARY HYPERTENSION

Hypertension may be due to essential/primary hypertension or secondary hypertension.
- Primary hypertension:
  - Does not have any underlying cause
  - Accounts for 90–95% of cases of hypertension
  - It is the result of interplay between genetic and environmental factors.
  - Tends to be familial in 30–40%.

- Secondary hypertension:
    - Accounts for 5–10% of the cases
    - High BP is due to specific underlying disorder

Secondary Hypertension[3]

It accounts for 5–10% of cases and is due to a specific underlying cause. Causes of secondary hypertension are as follows **(Table 3)**:

TABLE 3: Etiology of secondary hypertension.

Renal	Parenchymal diseases, renal cysts (polycystic kidney disease), obstructive uropathy, renal tumors
Renovascular	Arteriosclerotic, fibromuscular dysplasia
Adrenal	Pheochromocytoma, primary aldosteronism, Cushing syndrome, 17α-hydroxylase deficiency, 11β-hydroxylase deficiency, 11-hydroxysteroid dehydrogenase deficiency (licorice)
Coarctation of aorta	
Neurogenic	Psychogenic, diencephalic syndrome, familial dysautonomia, polyneuritis (acute porphyria, lead poisoning), acute increased intracranial pressure, acute spinal cord section
Drug induced	High-dose estrogens, adrenal steroids, decongestants, appetite suppressants, cyclosporine, tricyclic antidepressants, monoamine oxidase inhibitors, erythropoietin, nonsteroidal anti-inflammatory agents, cocaine
Endocrine	Hypothyroidism, hyperthyroidism, hypercalcemia, acromegaly
Preeclampsia/Eclampsia	
Mendelian forms	Liddle's syndrome, Gordon syndrome, Glucocorticoid remediable hypertension

Clinical Clues for Secondary Hypertension
- Early-onset hypertension (<30 years) in absence of risk factors
- No family history of hypertension
- Resistant hypertension
- Sudden deterioration in BP control
- Presenting with hypertensive urgency/emergency
- Clinical evaluation pointing toward any specific causes, e.g., pheochromocytoma, drug history, obstructive sleep apnea (OSA), and renal diseases.

RISKS OF HYPERTENSION ON HEALTH

- Globally, the prevalence of hypertension is 30–45% in adults with an estimated 1.13 billion affected in 2015.
- The prevalence increases with increasing age, >60% are affected in age group >60 years.[4]
- High BP is the leading risk factor attributing to 12.8% of global deaths, majority being due to CVDs, hemorrhagic strokes, or ischemic strokes. The interheart and interstroke studies report hypertension as an attributable risk for CVD and strokes at the tune of 17.9 and 34.6%, respectively.
- Latest data from India shows the prevalence in urban areas is 33.8% and in rural areas is 27.6% with an overall prevalence of 29.8%.[5]
- Hypertension-mediated organ damage (HMOD): HMOD refers to structural or functional changes in the arteries or end organs (heart, blood vessels, brain, kidney, and eyes) resulting from high BP. HMOD is a marker for asymptomatic CVD **(Tables 4 and 5)**.

TABLE 4: Hypertension-mediated organ dysfunction (HMOD).[5]

Cardiovascular disease	• Left ventricular hypertrophy • Left atrial enlargement • Diastolic dysfunction of LV (impaired relaxation) • Arrhythmias, especially atrial fibrillation • Heart failure with a preserved ejection fraction (HFpEF)
Vascular disease	• Carotid plaques and stenosis • Peripheral vascular disease (PVD) • Aortic dissection
Kidney disease	• Microalbuminuria/proteinuria • Chronic kidney disease
Cerebrovascular disease	• Transient ischemic attacks • Ischemic strokes • Hemorrhagic strokes • Cognitive impairment
Eye	Hypertensive retinopathy

TABLE 5: Evaluation of hypertension-mediated organ damage (HMOD).[4]

Cardiovascular disease	
ECG	• Left ventricular hypertrophy • Ischemic changes
2D echocardiography	• Left ventricular hypertrophy • Diastolic dysfunction • Systolic dysfunction

Continued

Continued

Vascular disease	
Carotid ultrasound	• Carotid intima-media thickness • Atherosclerotic plaques or stenosis
Ankle brachial index	Lower extremity artery disease
Carotid-femoral pulse wave velocity	Large artery stiffness
Kidney disease	
• Urine albumin: creatinine ratio • Serum creatinine • eGFR	Impaired renal function/chronic kidney disease
Renal ultrasound and Doppler	• Impaired renal function/chronic kidney disease • Suspected secondary renal hypertension
Cerebrovascular disease	
Brian CT scan/MRI	TIAs/ischemic or hemorrhagic strokes/cognitive decline
Eye	
Fundoscopy	Hypertensive retinopathy

(CT: computed tomography; ECG: electrocardiogram; eGFR: estimated glomerular filtration rate; MRI: magnetic resonance imaging; TIA: transient ischemic attack)

BLOOD PRESSURE MEASUREMENT

Accurate Blood Pressure Measurement

Blood pressure measurement is one of the simplest yet most erroneously performed medical procedures. It gives the clinician important data regarding the cardiac functionality, the peripheral circulation, target organ perfusion, etc. This part of the chapter attempts to elucidate accurate BP measurement procedure as a checklist, which the clinician can mentally mark off in daily practice so as to obtain correct BP reading.

The machines and methods that are available presently for BP measurement include the following mentioned below.

Mercury Sphygmomanometer (Fig. 1)

This is the traditional BP measurement machine, still very popularly used presently. It is very accurate in BP readings, but is largely operator-dependent. The concerns of mercury toxicity among the factory workers who manufacture this instrument have led to worldwide stoppage of further production of such instruments.

Measuring the cuff size is very important for accurate BP measurement **(Table 6)**.
- Most off-the-shelf monitors are stocked with a regular adult size cuff—may not be appropriate for everyone.

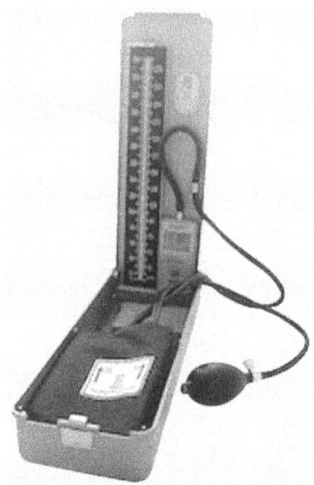

FIG. 1: Mercury sphygmomanometer.

TABLE 6: Cuff sizes.[6]

Cuff name	Bladder width	Bladder length	Mid arm circumference
Child	8	21	16 to <22 cm
Small arm	10	24	22 to <27 cm
Average arm	13	30	27 to <33 cm
Large arm	16	38	33 to <41 cm
Extra Large	17	43	41 to <52 cm

- Measure for accurate cuff size with a tape measure.
- Measure the arm from *Acromion to Olecranon*: At *the mid-point*—measure the mid arm circumference.
- Cuff size actually refers to the size of the bladder inside:
  - Cuff width should equal 40% of the arm circumference
  - Cuff length should equal 80% of the arm circumference
- Inappropriate cuff size:
  - If cuff used is too small → overestimation of BP
  - If cuff used is too wide → underestimation of BP

Automated Sphygmomanometer (Fig. 2)

With the mercury BP apparatus gradually being phased out, this electronic machine is gaining popularity. It is convenient to use, quick to measure, and can be used in both an office and home set up. The patients can also be taught its use, thereby allowing for home BP measurements. Arm (brachial artery) devices are more reliable. Wrist devices are not recommended.

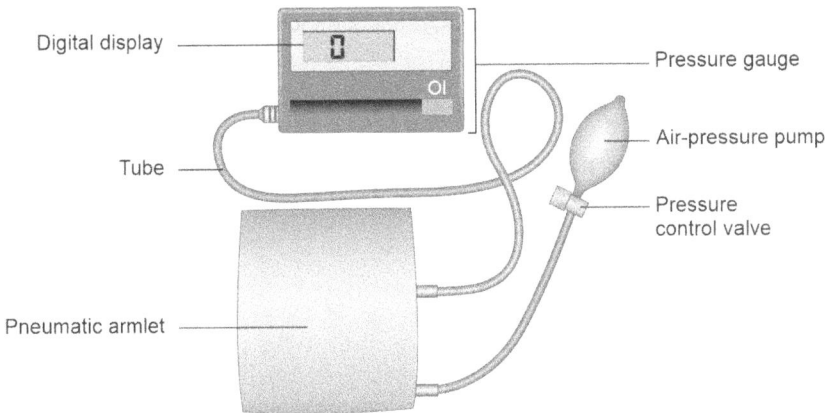

FIG. 2: Automated sphygmomanometer.

The error margin of the automated machines is still quite a bit and comparison with a mercury machine or an average of readings taken on the automated machine ensures the correct BP reading. The automated machines require calibration once in 6 months to a year, depending on the use.

Pneumatic Sphygmomanometer (Fig. 3)

Another alternative to the mercury BP apparatus is the pneumatic sphygmomanometer. It is quite accurate and very easy to use with low maintenance. Like the mercury instrument, it is very operator dependent and requires calibration.

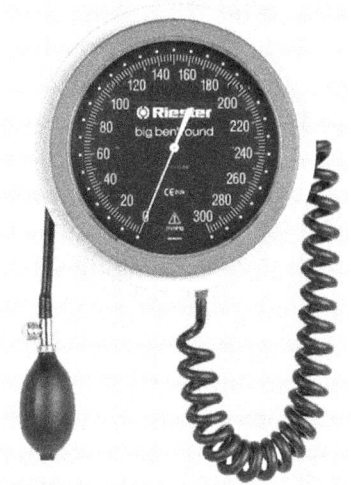

FIG. 3: Pneumatic sphygmomanometer.

Accurate Blood Pressure Check-Up (As a Procedural Checklist)

Instrument checklist
- *BP machine*: Mercury/pneumatic/electronic
- *Cuff size*: 70 cm (27.5 inches) for upper limb and it encircle 80% or more of the arm/thigh circumference.
- *Calibration*: Machines to be calibrated once in a 6 months

Patient checklist
- Preprocedure—no coffee/caffeinated drinks at least 1 hour prior
- Preprocedure—no alcohol consumption at least 12 hours prior
- Preprocedure—if the patient has just come to the clinician after climbing stairs or after a brisk walk, the clinician should wait for at least 20 minutes before measuring the BP
- Preprocedure—patient to empty bladder prior
- Preprocedure—allay anxiety of the patient (to minimize "white coat effect") by talking and reassuring the patient
- Preprocedure—ensure the patient has taken his/her antihypertensive that day as per the scheduled dose
- Ambient surroundings should be comfortable with adequate lighting and noise-free environment.
- Patient should be asked to remove tight clothing from the collar and or arm area.
- Patient position—seated with legs uncrossed (crossing of legs raise systolic pressure) and arms and back well supported (unsupported back raises the diastolic pressure)
- Expose the arm adequately for BP measurement (remove any clothing from the arm to avoid "tourniquet" effect during BP measurement.
- Do not measure BP in a paralyzed arm.

Procedure check list (Fig. 4 and Table 7)
- Do not converse during BP measurement.
- Patient's upper arm to be supported at his heart level, which is the midpoint of the sternum (if the upper arm is below the heart level the reading will be too high, if the upper arm is above the heart level, the reading will be too low).
- Locate the brachial artery pulsation in the antecubital fossa and apply the midline of the cuff above this pulsation.
- The lower edge of the cuff should be 2–3 cm from the antecubital fossa to allow space for the bell of the stethoscope.
- Inflate the cuff to 30 mm Hg above the point at which the radial pulse disappears (by palpatory method).
- Cuff to be deflated 2–3 mm Hg per second.
- The first Korotkoff sound heard (Phase I) is taken as the SBP and when the last Korotkoff sound disappears (Phase V) is taken as the DBP.
- Two readings in an interval of 1 minute are recommended and the average of the two is taken as the accurate BP.
- In the first visit, ensure BP is measured in both the arms to rule out coarctation of aorta.

CHAPTER 1 Defining and Measuring Blood Pressure

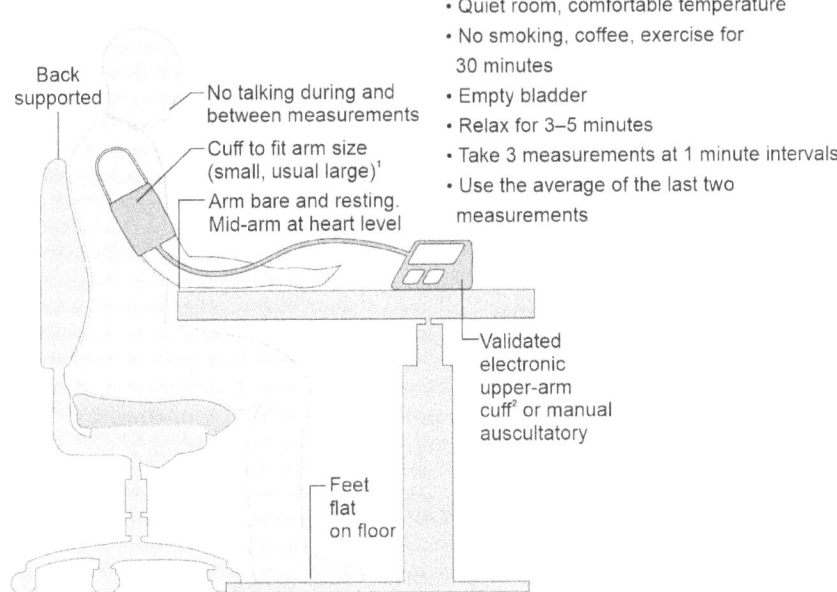

FIG. 4: Correct technique to measure blood pressure.

[1] For manual auscultatory devices the inflatable bladder of the cuff must cover 75–100% of the individual's arm circumference. For electronic devices use cuffs according to device instructions.
[2] See validated electronic devices lists at www.stridebp.org

Fallacies in Blood Pressure Measurement and Its Impact on the Readings

TABLE 7: Fallacies in blood pressure (BP) measurement and its impact on the readings.

Factor	Discrepancy in systolic/diastolic BP (mm Hg)
Talking	10/10
Distended bladder	15/10
Cuff over clothing	5–50/--
Cuff too small	10/2–8
Smoking within 1 hour of measurement	6–20/--
Paralyzed arm	2–5/--
Back unsupported	6–10/--
Arm unsupported, sitting	1–7/5–11
Arm unsupported, standing	6–8/--

Special Situations in Blood Pressure Measurement
- In an obese individual, BP cuff can be applied to the forearm and the radial reading can be taken.
- In a pregnant woman, the patient should be in a left lateral position and BP to be measured in the right upper arm.
- In an elderly individual, BP is to be measured in supine, sitting, and standing position to rule out orthostatic hypotension (drop >20 mm Hg of systolic pressure). Allow patient to stand for 2–3 minutes before BP is measured.

Diagnosing Hypertension
- Whenever possible, the diagnosis should not be made on a single office visit.
- Usually, two to three office visits at 1–4-week intervals (depending on the BP level) are required to confirm the diagnosis of hypertension.
- If value of SBP or DBP falls in different category, higher value should be used for diagnosis.
- The diagnosis might be made on a single visit, if BP is ≥180/110 mm Hg and there is evidence of HMOD.
- If possible, the diagnosis of hypertension should be confirmed by out-of-office BP measurement.

Out-of-Office Measurement of Blood Pressure
This can be done by two methods:
A. Ambulatory BP Measurement (ABPM)
B. Home BP Measurement (HBPM)

If feasible, should be used in confirming diagnosis of hypertension and is specifically indicated in masked hypertension, white-coat hypertension, guiding treatment, and its possible side effects.

Both have shown to be a better predictor for HMOD and cardiovascular morbidity and mortality.

A. Ambulatory Blood Pressure Measurement (Figs. 5A and B)
Automated procedure, which measures BP every 30 minutes over 24–48 hours (typically 50–75 readings in 24 hours).

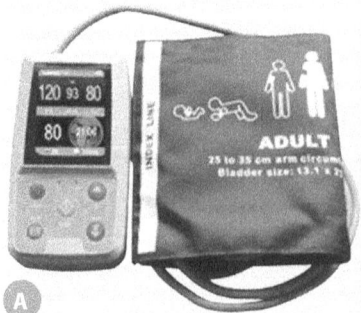
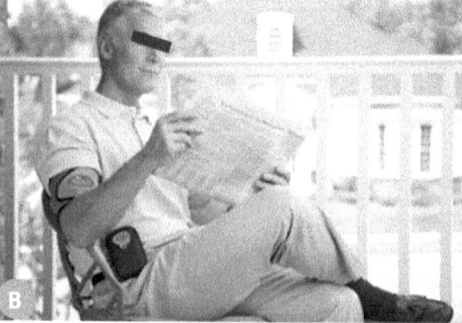

FIGS. 5A AND B: Ambulatory blood pressure measurement.

Procedural Details (Tables 8 to 10 and Fig. 6)
- Have the patient relax in a quiet room.
- Enter the patient's details, such as name and identification number, into the monitor.
- Measure BP in both arms.
- If the difference in SBP is <10 mm Hg, use the nondominant arm for monitoring.
- If the difference in SBP is ≥10 mm Hg, use the monitor on the arm with higher pressure.
- Select the appropriate cuff.
- Select the frequency of measurement (usually every 30 minutes).
- Inactivate the display to prevent the patient becoming distracted by the measurements.
- Give the patient written instructions.
- Show the patient how to remove and inactivate the monitor after 24 hours.
- Indications for ABPM:
  - To rule out white-coat hypertension
  - To identify masked hypertension
  - To identify "nondippers"

TABLE 8: Blood pressure cut-off as per ambulatory blood pressure (BP) measurements (ABPMs).[7]

Category	Systolic BP (mm Hg)	Diastolic BP (mm Hg)
24-hour mean	≥130	≥80
Day-time mean	≥135	≥85
Night-time mean	≥120	≥70

TABLE 9: Patterns of blood pressure (BP) variation on ambulatory blood pressure measurement (ABPM).[8,9]

Pattern	Definition	Interpretation
Dipping	Nocturnal BP fall of about 15% of day-time values	Physiological variation in normotensive and hypertensive patients
Nondipping	Absence of nocturnal fall of BP by atleast 10% of day-time values	• Nocturnal hypertension or obstructive sleep apnea • Independent predictor of CV and non-CV mortality
Extreme dipping	Marked fall of BP by >20% of day-time values	• Increased risks of strokes and CV mortality
Reverse dipping	Increase in the nocturnal BP readings to levels higher than daytime levels	• Nocturnal hypertension or obstructive sleep apnea • Independent predictor of CV and non-CV mortality
(CV: cardiovascular)		

TABLE 10: White-coat hypertension and masked hypertension (HTN).[10]

Pattern	Clinic BP	ABPM/ nonclinic BP	Pre-existing HTN	Interpretation
White-coat effect	Elevated	Normal	Yes	Often seen in patients with resistant HTN
White-coat hypertension (isolated clinic HTN)	Elevated	Normal	No	• Prevalence: 10–20% • More often in children, women, older adults • Cause of pseudoresistant HTN
Masked hypertension	Normal	Elevated	Yes/No	• Prevalence: 10–30% • Common in DM, CKD, OSA • Underestimates CV risk • Independent predictor of CV and non-CV mortality

(DM: diabetes mellitus; CKD: chronic kidney disease; CV: cardiovascular; OSA: obstructive sleep apnea)

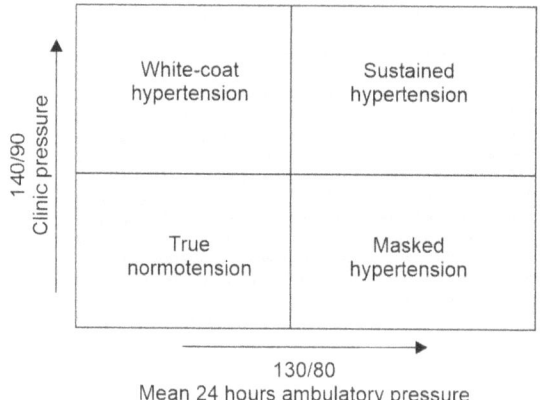

FIG. 6: Masked hypertension and white-coat hypertension.

- To monitor therapy
- To identify episodic hypotension/hypertension
- To identify autonomic neuropathy
- Advantages:
  - Greater reproducibility leads to accurate BP estimation.

- Helps in diagnosing borderline hypertension
- Helps to identify nocturnal hypertension
- Helps to diagnose and treat pregnancy-induced hypertension
- Antihypertensive dosages can be more tailor-made.
- Effect of antihypertensives on BP can be better ascertained.
- Reduces the placebo effect on BP
- Takes away the "white-coat" effect
- Can be useful for remote consultations, wherein the BP record can be electronically transmitted to the clinician.
  - Disadvantages:
    - Constant awareness of the cuff presence can lead to errors in BP readings
    - Can disturb the sleep of the patient, leading to alterations in BP
    - Cost-benefit ratio can matter for some patients.
  - *Interpretation*: Graphical record is generated and the peaks and the troughs are to be analyzed for diagnosis, treatment plan, and prognostication.

B. Home Blood Pressure Monitoring

- Automated machines used for measuring brachial artery pressure (arm pressure) are reliable. Wrist monitors are not recommended.
- Useful to rule out white-coat hypertension
- Useful pointers for HBPM:
  - Patient to sit 3–5 minutes in a comfortable chair before BP measurement.
  - Avoid caffeinated drinks/nicotine at least an hour before measurement.
  - Upper arm should be bare.
  - The arm should be supported on a firm surface at heart level.
  - The appropriate sized cuff should be used. It should snuggly fit the arm about half to one inch above the elbow crease.
  - Readings should be taken at 1-minute intervals. Two to three readings should be taken and average should be noted. This should be done twice a day for 7 days. The readings of the first day should be discarded and the remaining 12 readings should be averaged. HBPM is defined as the average of these 12 readings.
  - Extremes of readings to be brought to the attention of the attending clinician immediately.
  - Advantages:
    - Can detect "out-of-office" BP readings more accurately
    - Can identify white-coat hypertension
    - Can identify masked hypertension
    - Gives patients more active role in their BP management
    - Can increase treatment adherence
    - Can be useful for remote consultations, wherein the BP record can be electronically transmitted to the clinician
  - Disadvantages:
    - Accuracy of BP estimation cannot be quantified.
    - Can encourage self-dose adjustment

- Oscillometric devices may not work well in patients with atrial fibrillation or arrhythmias.
        - Need to be regularly calibrated against mercury sphygmomanometer
        - May not be possible in patients of cognitive or physical impairments
        - May aggravate conditions such as anxiety and obsessive compulsive disorder in some patients.
    o Special situations:
        - *Elderly*: BP variability tends to be high, and white-coat hypertension is common.
        - *Diabetics*: Tight BP control is important and home monitoring may help achieve this.
        - *Pregnancy*: The early detection of preeclampsia might be facilitated by HBPM.
        - *Chronic kidney disease*: BP may fluctuate a lot and home monitors help with management.
        - *Children*: White-coat hypertension occurs in children, and there are some data on normal home BP levels at different ages.

Central Aortic Blood Pressure

Central aortic pressure refers to pressure in the aorta, which reflects the actual BP without the "external" or "peripheral" interfering factors. CABP also reflects the actual aortic pressure, which is very significant for prognostication and deciding therapy. It is measured by cardiac catheterization, which being an invasive procedure, carries with its a set of risks and complications. Recently, a number of noninvasive methods have been devised for measuring the CABP, such as recording wave forms over radial, brachial, and carotid arteries and comparing them to the sphygmomanometer. However, these BP measurements are time-consuming and the machines are not widely available.

Screening for Hypertension

As hypertension is predominantly asymptomatic, it is important for a structured screening program for early diagnosis.

All adults (starting at age of 18 years) should be screened as below **(Table 11)**.

TABLE 11: Frequency for office blood pressure (BP) screening.

Office BP	Screening period
Healthy with BP <120/80 mm Hg	Every 5 years or more frequently as indicated
Normal BP 120–129/80–84 mm Hg	Every 3 years or more frequently as indicated
High normal 130–139/85–89 mm Hg	Every year

SUMMARY

- Optimal BP is SBP <120 mm Hg and DBP <80 mm Hg.
- Indian Guidelines of Hypertension classify hypertension as SBP ≥140 mm Hg or DBP ≥90 mm Hg.
- Hypertension is primary/essential (without a cause) in 90–95% of cases. In certain cases, workup for ruling our secondary/treatable causes should be done.
- All hypertension patients should be screened for HMOD.
- The measurement of BP should be done accurately with an accurate BP machine and an appropriately sized cuff.
- HBPM and ABPM should be done in special situations to diagnose masked hypertension, white-coat hypertension, and resistant hypertension.

MULTIPLE CHOICE QUESTIONS

1. Which of the following is not a cause for drug induced hypertension?
   A. Cyclosporine
   B. Decongestants
   C. Appetite suppressants
   D. All of the above

2. Which of the following is a direct cause for secondary hypertension?
   A. Fibromuscular dysplasia
   B. Megaloblastic anemia
   C. Dyslipidemia
   D. None of the above

3. Which of the following values is a diagnostic criteria for hypertension?
   A. ABPM night-time mean 130 mm Hg systolic and/or 80 mm Hg diastolic
   B. ABPM day-time mean 130 mm Hg systolic and/or 80 mm Hg diastolic
   C. HBPM systolic 135 mm Hg and/or diastolic 85 mm Hg
   D. Office BP 145 mm Hg systolic and/or 95 mm Hg diastolic

4. Which of the following endocrine anomaly is not a cause for secondary hypertension?
   A. Acromegaly
   B. Hypothyroidism
   C. Hyperprolactinemia
   D. Cushing syndrome

5. The following are false statements, except:
   A. White-coat effect is elevated clinic and normal ABPM in normotensive patients
   B. Masked hypertension is normal clinic and normal ABPM in hypertensive patients
   C. White-coat effect is elevated clinic and normal ABPM in hypertensive patients
   D. Masked hypertension is elevated clinic and normal ABPM in normotensive patients

Answers

1—D 2—A 3—C 4—C 5—C

REFERENCES

1. Ministry of Health and Family Welfare Government of India. (2016). Standard treatment guidelines. Hypertension screening, diagnosis, assessment, and management of primary hypertension in adults in India. [online] Available from: http://clinicalestablishments.gov.in/WriteReadData/6591.pdf. [Last accessed December, 2022].
2. Huang QF, Yang WY, Asayama K, Zhang ZY, Thijs L, Li Y, et al. Ambulatory blood pressure monitoring to diagnose and manage hypertension. Hypertension. 2021;77(2):254-64.
3. Hegde S, Aeddula NR. Secondary hypertension. In: StatPearls. Treasure Island (FL): StatPearls Publishing; 2022.
4. Schmieder RE. End organ damage in hypertension. Dtsch Arztebl Int. 2010;107(49):866-73.
5. Oh JS, Lee CH, Park JI, Park HK, Hwang JK. Hypertension-mediated organ damage and long-term cardiovascular outcomes in asian hypertensive patients without prior cardiovascular disease. J Korean Med Sci. 2020;35(48):e400.
6. Palatini P, Asmar R. Cuff challenges in blood pressure measurement. J Clin Hypertens (Greenwich). 2018;20(7):1100-3.
7. O'Brien E, White WB, Parati G, Dolan E. Ambulatory blood pressure monitoring in the 21st century. J Clin Hypertens (Greenwich). 2018;20(7):1108-11.
8. Redon J, Lurbe E. Nocturnal blood pressure versus nondipping pattern what do they mean? Hypertension. 2008;51(1):41-2.
9. Routledge F, McFetridge-Durdle J. Nondipping blood pressure patterns among individuals with essential hypertension: a review of the literature. Eur J Cardiovasc Nurs. 2007;6(1):9-26.
10. Stergiou GS, Asayama K, Thijs L, Kollias A, Niiranen TJ, Hozawa A, et al. Prognosis of white-coat and masked hypertension international database of home blood pressure in relation to cardiovascular outcome. Hypertension. 2014;63(4):675-82.

SUGGESTED READINGS

1. Lewington S, Clarke R, Qizilbash N, Peto R, Collins R; Prospective Studies Collaboration. Age-specific relevance of usual blood pressure to vascular mortality: a meta-analysis of individual data for one million adults in 61 prospective studies. Lancet. 2002;360(9349):1903-13.
2. Rapsomaniki E, Timmis A, George J, Pujades-Rodriguez M, Shah AD, Denaxas S, et al. 2014 Blood pressure and incidence of twelve cardiovascular diseases: lifetime risks, healthy life-years lost, and age-specific associations in 1.25 million people. Lancet. 2014;383(9932):1899-911.
3. Whelton PK, Carey RM, Aronow WS, Casey DE Jr, Collins KJ, Dennison Himmelfarb C, et al. 2017 ACC/AHA/AAPA/ABC/ACPM/AGS/APhA/ASH/ASPC/NMA/PCNA guideline for the prevention, detection, evaluation, and management of high blood pressure in adults. A report of the American College of Cardiology/American Heart Association Task Force on Clinical Practice Guidelines. J Am Coll Cardiol. 2018;71(19):e127-248.

4. Shah S, Munjal YP, Kamath SA, Wander GS, Mehta N, Mukherjee S, et al. Indian guidelines on Hypertension IV (I.G.H. IV). J Assoc Physicians India. 2019;67(9):1-48.
5. Williams B, Mancia G, Spiering W, Agabiti Rosei E, Azizi M, Burnier M, et al. 2018 ESC/ESH Guidelines for the management of arterial hypertension. The Task Force for the management of arterial hypertension of the European Society of Cardiology (ESC) and the European Society of Hypertension (ESH). Eur Heart J. 2018;39(33):3021-104.
6. Harianto H, Valente M, Hoetomo S, Anpalahan M. The clinical utility of ambulatory blood pressure monitoring (ABPM): a review. Curr Hypertens Rev. 2014;10(4): 189-204.

CHAPTER 2

Clinical Features and Investigations

Nikesh Jain

CLINICAL EVALUATION

- Patients with hypertension (HTN) are usually asymptomatic—diagnosed during routine check-up or during evaluation of other illness.
- Patient may have following symptoms/signs due to HTN or hypertension-mediated organ damage (HMOD) or underlying secondary cause—headache, dizziness, chest pain, palpitations, breathlessness, edema feet, nocturia, claudication, blurring of vision, and stroke.
- HMOD:
  - It refers to structural or functional changes in arteries or end organs (heart, blood vessels, brain, eyes, and kidney) caused by an elevated blood pressure (BP).
  - It is common in severe or long-standing HTN, but can be found in less severe cases and increasingly found in asymptomatic cases as initial presentation.
  - HMOD increases cardiovascular (CV) risk and risk increases linearly when multiple organs are involved.
  - HMOD can be reversed with early and strict control of HTN. If present for a long-time, it cannot be reversed but progression can be delayed with control of HTN.

Patient with HTN should be clinically evaluated as follows.

HISTORY

It should be directed toward following three factors **(Table 1)**:

TABLE 1: History taking of patient with hypertension.[1]

Current medical history and risk factor evaluation:
• *Details about HTN*: Duration of HTN, current and previous BP recordings, current and past medicines for HTN, including compliance to treatment, previous HTN in eclampsia/preeclampsia

Continued

Continued

- *Past history of:* Medical/surgical illness and ongoing treatment for any illness, use of medications such as OC pills, herbal remedies, licorice (Jethimadh), NSAIDs, corticosteroids, nasal decongestants, etc.
- *Family history of:* HTN or other risk factors—Diabetes, dyslipidemia, cardiovascular (CV) diseases, premature CAD, and renal diseases.
- *Lifestyle and other risk factors:* Exercise level, weight changes, dietary habits—salt intake, smoking, alcohol consumption, recreational drug use, sleep pattern—obstructive sleep apnea, history of erectile dysfunction, early menopause
- *Additional CV risk factor evaluation:* Diabetes, dyslipidemia, exertional angina/breathlessness, claudication, and stroke

History and symptoms of HMOD and associated clinical conditions influencing CV risk:
- *Heart:* Chest pain, breathlessness on exertion, edema feet, syncope, palpitations (atrial fibrillation), prior myocardial infarction/revascularization, heart failure
- *Brain:* Headache, vertigo, syncope, prior TIA/stroke, carotid revascularization, early cognitive impairment/dementia
- *Eyes:* Blurring of vision, floaters, retinal therapies/evaluation documenting hypertensive changes
- *Kidney:* Polyuria, nocturia, recurrent UTI, familial disease (polycystic kidney disease), past creatinine/renal Doppler parameters
- *Peripheral arteries:* Claudication, nonhealing wound/gangrene, peripheral revascularization, and erectile dysfunction

Look for secondary causes of HTN:
- History suggestive of secondary HTN and its causes (discussed in Chapter 1)

(CAD: coronary artery disease; HMOD: hypertension-mediated organ damage; HTN: hypertension; NSAID: nonsteroidal anti-inflammatory drug; OC: oral contraceptive; TIA: transient ischemic attack; UTI: urinary tract infection)

PHYSICAL EXAMINATION

It provides information regarding associated comorbidities, HMOD, and secondary causes of HTN **(Table 2)**.

TABLE 2: Comprehensive clinical examination.[1]

- Diagnosing HTN:
  - Correct method of checking office BP (discussed in Chapter 1)
  - Take BP in both arms and lower limb
  - Take supine and standing BP
- Body habitus:
  - Weight, height, and BMI
  - Waist circumference

Continued

Continued

- Look for HMOD:
  - *Heart*: Pulse (arrhythmias—AF), location and character of apex beat (concentric LVH), 3rd/4th heart sound, and murmurs
  - *Peripheral arterial disease*: Equality of peripheral pulses, bruits—renal/carotid, ankle brachial index, measuring BP in both arms, arteriopathic changes in limbs—cold, loss of hair, and shiny skin
  - *Nervous system*: Residual motor/sensory deficits and cognitive status
  - *Fundoscopy*: To evaluate hypertensive retinopathy
  - *Abdominal system*: Palpable aortic pulsations
- *Secondary hypertension:* Look for specific signs indicating specific disease/syndrome—
  - *Coarctation of aorta*: Radiofemoral delay, BP in upper limbs > lower limbs, murmur, and bruits
  - *Renal bruit*: Atherosclerotic renal occlusion, fibromuscular dysplasia (FMD), and Takayasu's disease
  - *Palpable abdominal mass*: Palpable kidneys (polycystic kidney disease), adrenal/renal tumors
  - Features of Cushing syndrome
  - *Features of thyroid disease*: Hypo-/hyperthyroidism
  - *Café-au-lait patches of neurofibromatosis*: Pheochromocytoma

(AF: atrial fibrillation; BMI: body mass index; BP: blood pressure; HMOD: hypertension-mediated organ damage; HTN: hypertension; LVH: left ventricular hypertrophy)

INVESTIGATIONS

Essential Hypertension (Table 3)

TABLE 3: Investigations in a case of essential hypertension.[1]

- Routine investigations—to guide treatment and evaluate additional CV risk:
  - Hemoglobin and hematocrit
  - BUN, creatinine, and eGFR
  - Serum sodium and potassium
  - Fasting lipid profile
  - FBS, PPBS, and HbA1c
  - Urine routine/microscopy and urine dipstick test for protein
- To diagnose and assess severity of HMOD:
  - Heart:
    - ECG: LVH, arrhythmias (AF), associated changes—old MI
    - 2D ECHO: LVH with repolarization changes, systolic and diastolic function, associated abnormalities—valvular heart disease

Continued

- Kidney:
  - *Urine albumin creatinine ratio*: To quantify albuminuria
  - *USG with Doppler*: To look for kidney size, structural kidney disease—obstructive uropathy and atherosclerotic renal artery stenosis
- Peripheral vascular involvement:
  - Ankle Brachial Index
  - Lower limb Doppler
  - CT angiography if clinically required
- Evaluation of aorta:
  - Imaging: USG (pulse wave velocity: PWV—index of aortic stiffness and arteriosclerosis)
  - Computed tomography scan for atherosclerotic changes and aneurysm
- Neurological evaluation:
  - CT/MRI: History of CVA, cognitive decline
  - Carotid Doppler: To detect plaques/stenosis in patients with CVA
  - Cognitive function testing
- *Fundoscopy*: To look for hypertensive retinopathy changes

(AF: atrial fibrillation; BUN: blood urea nitrogen; CT: computed tomography; CV: cardiovascular; CVA: cerebrovascular accident; ECG: electrocardiography; eGFR: estimated glomerular filtration rate; FBS: fasting blood sugar; HbA1c: glycosylated hemoglobin; HTN: hypertension; LVH: left ventricular hypertrophy; MI: myocardial infarction; MRI: magnetic resonance imaging; PPBS: post-prandial blood sugar; USG: ultrasonography; HMOD: hypertension-mediated organ damage)

Secondary Hypertension (Table 4)

TABLE 4: Investigations in a suspected case of secondary hypertension (HTN) should be directed as per findings on clinical evaluation.[2]

Renal and renovascular causes	*Urine routine/microscopy*: Parenchymal diseases
	USG or CT: Renal/adrenal tumors, polycystic kidney disease
	Doppler/CT angiography: Renal artery stenosis—atherosclerotic/FMD/Takayasu's
Coarctation of aorta	2D echocardiography and CT angiography
Cushing syndrome	Dexamethasone suppression test
	Rule out steroid-induced Cushing syndrome
Primary aldosteronism	Plasma aldosterone to renin activity ratio, saline infusion test, 24-hour urine aldosterone level
Pheochromocytoma	24-hour urine metanephrine and normetanephrine levels
Thyroid/parathyroid disorders	T3, T4, TSH, PTH, imaging: USG/nuclear scan
Obstructive sleep apnea	Sleep study

Continued

Drug related	*Drug screening*: NSAID, recreational drug use, sympathomimetics, corticosteroids, herbal medicines, OC pills, cyclosporine, tacrolimus,
(CT: computed tomography; FMD: fibromuscular dysplasia; NSAID: nonsteroidal anti-inflammatory drug; OC: oral contraceptive; PTH: parathyroid hormone; TSH: thyroid stimulating hormone; T3: triiodothyronine; T4: thyroxine; USG: ultrasonography)	

SUMMARY

- Patients with HTN are usually asymptomatic and typically diagnosed during routine checkup or evaluation for other illness.
- HMOD refers to structural or functional changes in arteries or end organs such as heart, blood vessels, brain, eyes and kidney caused by an elevated BP.
- Clinical evaluation is aimed at diagnosing HTN by taking history and symptoms, comprehensive physical examination and investigations.
- History taking in a patient with HTN should be directed toward the following: Details about HTN, past history, family history, lifestyle and other risk factors, CV risk factor evaluation, history and symptoms of HMOD and associated clinical conditions influencing CV risk as well as looking for secondary causes of HTN.
- Physical examination is aimed at the following: Diagnosing HTN, presence of other comorbidities, evaluation of HMOD and secondary HTN.
- Investigations in a case of essential HTN include—routine investigations, Investigations to diagnose and assess severity of HMOD
- Investigations in a case for secondary HTN should be based on findings of above clinical evaluation.

MULTIPLE CHOICE QUESTIONS

1. Which of the following is a false statement?
   A. HMOD can occur in patients with prolonged duration of HTN or even in less severe cases
   B. Once established HMOD can be completely reversed with HTN control even if in advanced stage
   C. Strict control of HTN can reverse or slow progression of HMOD
   D. All patients of HTN should be evaluated for HMOD
2. Which of the following is an investigation for pheochromocytoma?
   A. USG kidney with Doppler
   B. Dexamethasone suppression test
   C. 24-hour urine metanephrine and normetanephrine levels
   D. 24-hour urine aldosterone levels

3. Which of the following is not a clue for secondary HTN?
   A. Family history of HTN
   B. Sudden deterioration of HTN control
   C. Resistant HTN
   D. Early onset (<30 years) of HTN

4. Following are cardiovascular sign caused due to HMOD, except:
   A. Arrhythmias
   B. 3rd/4th heart sound gallop
   C. Early diastolic murmur—due to A1
   D. Absent apex beat

5. Which of the following is an investigation for Cushing syndrome?
   A. USG kidney
   B. 24-hour urine metanephrine and normetanephrine levels
   C. Drug screening for corticosteroids
   D. Saline infusion test

Answers

1—B   2—C   3—A   4—D   5—C

REFERENCES

1. Unger T, Borghi C, Charchar F, Khan NA, Poulter NR, Prabhakaran D, et al. 2020 International Society of Hypertension Global Hypertension Practice Guidelines. Hypertension. 2020;75(6):1334-57.
2. Rossi GP, Bisogni V, Rossitto G, Maiolino G, Cesari M, Zhu R, et al. Practice recommendations for diagnosis and treatment of the most common forms of secondary hypertension. High Blood Press Cardiovasc Prev. 2020;27(6):547-60.

SUGGESTED READINGS

1. Shah SN, Munjal YP, Kamath SA, Wander GS, Mehta N, Mukherjee S, et al. Indian guidelines on hypertension IV. J Assoc Physicians India. 2019;67(9):8-46.
2. Williams B, Mancia G, Spiering W, Agabiti Rosei E, Azizi M, Burnier M, et al. 2018 ESC/ESH guidelines for the management of arterial hypertension. Eur Heart J. 2018;39(33):3021-104.
3. Hinderliter AL, Lin FC, Viera LA, Olsson E, Klein JL, Viera AJ. Hypertension-mediated organ damage in masked hypertension. J Hypertens. 2022;40(4):811-8.
4. Flack JM, Adekola B. Blood pressure and the new ACC/AHA hypertension guide. Trends Cardiovasc Med. 2020;30(3):160-4.
5. Seravalle G, Grassi G. Sleep apnea and hypertension. High Blood Press Cardiovasc Prev. 2022;29(1):23-31.
6. Ferdinand KC, Nasser SA. Management of essential hypertension. Cardiol Clin. 2017;35(2):231-46.
7. Rimoldi SF, Scherrer U, Messerli FH. Secondary arterial hypertension: when, who, and how to screen? Eur Heart J. 2014;35(19):1245-54.

CHAPTER 3

Lifestyle Management

Ruchit Shah

INTRODUCTION

Hypertension is a lifestyle disease. Lifestyle change is the cornerstone of hypertension management. Lifestyle changes should be emphasized in each and every patient of hypertension, even if drug therapy is initiated.

Lifestyle changes should be highlighted in the population at large, in normotensive people, and hypertensive patients. The idea should be to inculcate a healthy lifestyle from childhood. A program which integrates healthcare workers, children, parents, schools, communities, and patients as a whole should be developed.

There is sufficient evidence to prove that lifestyle changes reduce blood pressure (BP) and improve cardiovascular (CV) outcomes. However, it should not delay drug treatment initiation in patients with end-organ damage or high CV risk.

Patient education regarding the disease pattern, lifestyle changes, drug compliance, and prevention of complications with hypertension is important. Every follow-up visit for hypertension should include reiteration of lifestyle changes.

LIFESTYLE INTERVENTIONS (TABLE 1)

Diet
- It is important to read and understand food labels.
- The diet should be low calorie and low fat.
- Saturated fats, total fats, and cholesterol should be reduced.
- Carbohydrate intake should be reduced.
- Low carbohydrate intake is associated with a lower mortality and stroke.
- The diet should include a high content of fresh fruits, green vegetables, fibers, sprouts, and roots.
- Whole grain intake in the form of cereals, bread, rice, and pasta should be increased.
- Walnuts, almonds, and hazelnuts may be added.
- A high protein intake in the form of eggs, poultry, low fat dairy products, meat, and plant protein is associated with BP reduction.

TABLE 1: Lifestyle interventions.[1,2]

Intervention	Recommendation	Systolic BP reduction
Diet (DASH)	Fruits, vegetables, whole cereals, low fat dairy products, less saturated, and total fats	8–14 mm Hg
Sodium	Sodium <2.4 g/day (salt <6 g/day)	2–8 mm Hg
Alcohol	Total abstinence preferred. <1 drink/day (F) and <2 drinks/day (M)	2–4 mm Hg
Weight	Maintain BMI 20–25 kg/m^2	5–20 mm Hg for 10 kg weight loss
Exercises	Aerobic-exercises: 30 min/day for 5–7 days a week	4–9 mm Hg
Smoking	Do not start smoking; if started quit smoking. Tobacco abstinence	

(BMI: body mass index; DASH: Dietary Approaches to Stop Hypertension)

- Avoid red meat.
- Fish is rich in omega-3 fatty acids which is beneficial.
- Consumption of sweets, sugar sweetened beverages, and carbonated drinks should be reduced.
- Use of rapeseed or flaxseed oil and olive oil should be encouraged.
- Fried food and junk food should be avoided.
- Vegetarians have a high intake of whole grains, fruits, vegetables, fibers, and low saturated fats which is healthy.

Dietary Sodium

- Worldover, dietary sodium intake is 3.5–5.5 g/day (9–12 g of salt/day). The mean salt intake in India is 9–14 g/day. It is advisable to reduce the dietary sodium intake to <2.4 g/day (<6 g of salt/day). One flattened teaspoon is equivalent to 5 g of salt. There is data to suggest that increased sodium intake, leads to rise in BP, and sodium restriction leads to reduction in BP. The effect of sodium restriction is well seen in blacks, old age, diabetics, metabolic syndrome, and chronic kidney disease (CKD) patients. It may also reduce the number of antihypertensives.
- One must avoid extra salt, processed foods, salt-preserved foods (pickles, chutneys, ketchups, papads, canned food, namkeens, and chips), French fries, foods containing baking powder, pizzas, Chinese, readymade soups, bakery products (breads, biscuits, and cakes), cheese, peanut butter, salted butter, and high salt-containing foods.

Potassium

- Increased potassium intake can cause BP reduction (avoid excessive potassium especially with drugs that cause hyperkalemia). Fresh fruits and vegetables are a rich source of potassium.
- Magnesium and calcium intake should be increased.
- DASH (Dietary Approaches to Stop Hypertension) and Mediterranean diet are the recommended diet plans. The diet plans vary according to

the eating habits of the individual and it is best to customize it for every patient with the help of a certified dietician.

Alcohol

- There is a correlation between alcohol consumption, hypertension, and CV risk, hence total abstinence is preferred. Moderation of alcohol intake is suggested, i.e., <2 drinks/day for men and <1 drink/day for women. Each unit equals to 125 mL of wine, 250 mL of beer, and 25 mL of spirits. However, depending on brand, concentration, type of alcohol, and country in which it is served, units may differ. Even people who are light or moderate drinkers may benefit from reduction in alcohol intake. Binge drinking must be strongly avoided. It is advisable to have alcohol-free days.
- *Coffee contains caffeine:* Caffeine is known to raise BP, but may be associated with CV benefits. Green and black tea may also have mild BP-lowering effect.

Weight

- Overweight and obesity are associated with raised BP, increased CV morbidity, and mortality. Weight reduction is associated with decreased BP and decreased CV events. Visceral obesity and waist circumference reduction confer significant benefit. Weight reduction by every kilogram reduces the BP by 1 mm Hg. Avoid body mass index (BMI) >30 kg/m^2 and waist circumference >102 in men and >88 cm in women. It is best to have BMI 20–25 kg/m^2 and waist circumference <94 cm for men and <80 cm for women. Weight reduction should involve physical exercises, dietary changes, and motivational counseling. It should be maintained over a long period of time. Antiobesity drugs and bariatric surgery are options available for morbid obesity.

Physical Activity

- It is advisable to do moderate-intensity dynamic aerobic exercise (swimming, walking, jogging, and cycling) for 30 minutes a day for 5–7 days a week. Resistance exercises may be added for 2–3 days a week. The intensity of exercises can be gradually increased to 300 minutes of moderate intensity or 150 minutes of vigorous exercises. Isometric exercises such as weight lifting can raise BP and are better avoided.

Smoking

- Active and passive smoking is a major risk factor for CV diseases and cancer. Quit smoking is the single most important thing which can be done for protecting CV health. Stopping tobacco products is associated with decreased CV risk and events including stroke, myocardial infarction, and peripheral arterial disease. Varenicline (better than bupropion) and combination nicotine replacement therapy along with behavioral therapy and counseling increase the success of quitting smoking. E-cigarettes are now available and are harmful, hence needs to be discouraged.

Yoga and Meditation

- Regular practice of yoga and meditation is a stress reliever. It reduces BP by 2-6 mm Hg, heart rate, waist circumference, and lipid profile. These are metabolic factors which influence long-term morbidity and mortality. A meta-analysis showed practice of yoga which contains postures, breath control, and meditation brought about a significant reduction in BP. Poses with forward bend and head supported, *Shavasana*, conscious breathing (*Pranayama*), meditation, and relaxation techniques have a beneficial effect on BP. Handstand poses (*Adho Mukha Vrksasana*), headstand poses (*Shirshasana*), and poses that compress the diaphragm should be avoided by hypertensive patients.

SUMMARY

- Lifestyle changes are the cornerstone of treatment of hypertension and should be advised to every patient irrespective of drug therapy.
- DASH diet plan suggests eating a diet rich in vegetables, fresh fruits, whole grain, fibers, high protein, fish, and low fat dairy products. Saturated and total fats should be reduced.
- Sodium intake should be restricted to <2.4 g/day (salt <6 g/day).
- Stop tobacco and smoking.
- Moderation of alcohol intake, with a preference for abstinence.
- Weight reduction and maintain BMI 20-25 kg/m^2
- Aerobic physical activity for 30 minutes/day for 5-7 days a week.

MULTIPLE CHOICE QUESTIONS

1. What is the recommended salt intake for a hypertensive patient?
    A. 3 g/day
    B. 6 g/day
    C. 8 g/day
    D. 10 g/day

2. The DASH diet plan constitutes all, except:
    A. Low fat dairy
    B. Low saturated fats
    C. High carbohydrate diet
    D. High protein diet

3. The recommended BMI to reduce CV risk is:
    A. <20 kg/m^2
    B. <25 kg/m^2
    C. <30 kg/m^2
    D. <40 kg/m^2

4. The following therapies should be used in order to quit smoking, except:
   A. Combination nicotine replacement therapy
   B. E-cigarettes
   C. Behavior therapy
   D. Counseling

5. The following physical activity is recommended for hypertensive patients, except:
   A. Brisk walking for 30 minutes
   B. Weight lifting
   C. Resistance exercises
   D. High-intensity interval training

Answers

1—B   2—C   3—B   4—B   5—B

REFERENCES

1. Eckel RH, Jakicic JM, Ard JD, de Jesus JM, Houston Miller N, Hubbard VS, et al. 2013 AHA/ACC guideline on lifestyle management to reduce cardiovascular risk: a report of the American College of Cardiology/American Heart Association Task Force on Practice Guidelines. Circulation. 2014;129(25 Suppl 2):S76-99.
2. Blumenthal JA, Hinderliter AL, Smith PJ, Mabe S, Watkins LL, Craighead L, et al. Effects of lifestyle modification on patients with resistant hypertension: results of the triumph randomized clinical trial. J Clin Hypertens (Greenwich). 2022.

SUGGESTED READINGS

1. He LI, Wei WR, Can Z. Effects of 12-week brisk walking training on exercise blood pressure in elderly patients with essential hypertension: a pilot study. Clin Exp Hypertens. 2018;40(7):673-9.
2. Prasertsri P, Phoemsapthawee J, Kuamsub S, Poolpol K, Boonla O. Effects of long-term regular continuous and intermittent walking on oxidative stress, metabolic profile, heart rate variability, and blood pressure in older adults with hypertension. J Environ Public Health. 2022;2022:5942947.
3. Saco-Ledo G, Valenzuela PL, Ruiz-Hurtado G, Ruilope LM, Lucia A. Exercise reduces ambulatory blood pressure in patients with hypertension: A systematic review and meta-analysis of randomized controlled trials. J Am Heart Assoc. 2020;9(24):e018487.
4. Ratchford SM, Broxterman RM, La Salle DT, Kwon OS, Park SY, Hopkins PN, et al. Salt restriction lowers blood pressure at rest and during exercise without altering peripheral hemodynamics in hypertensive individuals. Am J Physiol Heart Circ Physiol. 2019;317(6):H1194-202.
5. Garfinkle MA. Salt and essential hypertension: pathophysiology and implications for treatment. J Am Soc Hypertens. 2017;11(6):385-91.

CHAPTER 4

Drug Therapy

Ruchit Shah, Nihar Mehta

- **4.1:** Angiotensin-converting Enzyme Inhibitors, Angiotensin Receptor Blockers, and Renin Inhibitors
  Ruchit Shah
- **4.2:** Calcium Channel Blockers
  Ruchit Shah
- **4.3:** Diuretics
  Amjad Khan
- **4.4:** Beta-blockers
  Ruchit Shah
- **4.5:** Other Drugs
  Sudhiranjan Dash Choudhury, Ruchit Shah
- **4.6:** Newer Therapies for Systemic Hypertension: Renal Denervation Therapy and Baroreceptor Activation Therapy
  Ruchit Shah, Srinivasan Narayanan

4.1 Angiotensin-converting Enzyme Inhibitors, Angiotensin Receptor Blockers, and Renin Inhibitors

Ruchit Shah

MECHANISM OF ACTION

Renin-angiotensin-aldosterone system (RAAS) is activated in response to low blood volume, low blood pressure (BP), and lack of sodium. With increase in salt intake, ideally RAAS should be suppressed. Activation of the RAAS plays an important role in endothelial dysfunction, vascular remodeling, and hypertension. In hypertension with high sodium intake, any degree of RAAS activation should be suppressed. The risk of developing HTN increases with increasing levels of serum aldosterone.

Renin is formed in the juxtaglomerular cells of the kidney. It is released in response to low blood volume, low BP, and lack of sodium (Na). Renin helps in converting angiotensinogen to angiotensin I in the liver. Angiotensin-converting enzyme (ACE), which is present on the endothelial lining of the lungs, helps in converting angiotensin I to angiotensin II. ACE also causes breakdown of bradykinin. Angiotensin II acts on AT1 receptor. This causes aldosterone release leading to Na and water retention, potassium (K) excretion, and raised BP.

The sites of action of various classes of drugs are shown in **Flowchart 1**.

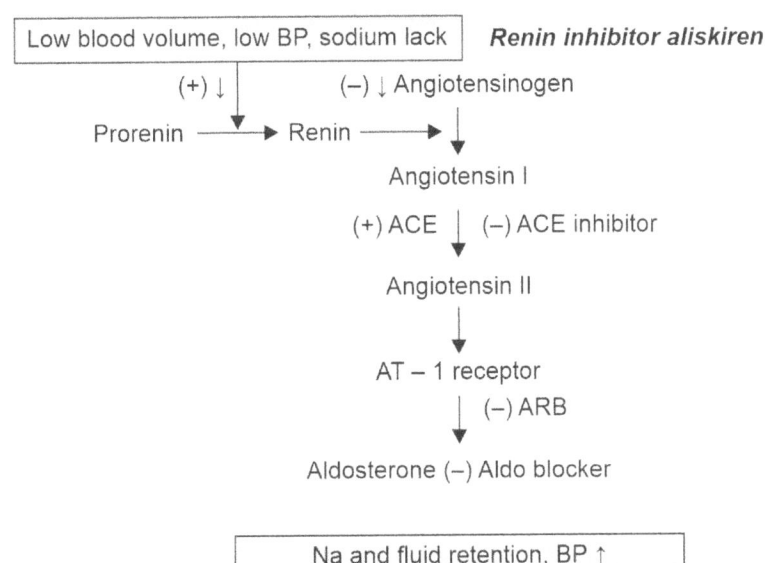

FLOWCHART 1: The sites of action of various classes of drugs.
(ACE: angiotensin-converting enzyme; ARB: angiotensin receptor blockers; BP: blood pressure)

PATHOGENIC PROPERTIES (TABLE 1)

TABLE 1: Pathogenic properties.[1,2]

Angiotensin II	ACE inhibitors
Heart: Myocardial hypertrophy and interstitial fibrosis	↓LVH, ↓wall stress, improves postinfarct remodeling
Coronary arteries: Endothelial dysfunction, ↑oxidative stress, ↑LDL uptake, ↑inflammatory response → atheroma formation	↓Atherogenesis, ↓thrombosis ↓sudden cardiac arrest
Kidney: ↑intraglomerular pressure, glomerular fibrosis, protein leak, and Na reabsorption	↓Proteinuria
Adrenal: ↑aldosterone – Na and water retention, K excretion; cardiac fibrosis, endothelial dysfunction	
↑Fibrinogen	
↑Adrenergic tone → ↑norepinephrine release → vasoconstriction	Antiadrenergic, vagomimetic, peripheral vasodilatation → ↓BP
Bradykinin degradation	↑bradykinin (?protects endothelium and ↓BP)

(BP: blood pressure; LDL: low-density lipoprotein; LVH: left ventricular hypertrophy; Na: sodium; K: potassium)

ANGIOTENSIN II RECEPTORS—AT-1, AT-2, AND AT-4 (TABLE 2)

TABLE 2: Angiotensin II receptors—AT-1, AT-2, and AT-4.[3]

AT-1	Vasoconstriction, endothelial dysfunction
	Stimulation of contraction
	Myocyte hypertrophy, fibrosis
	↑Aldosterone → antinatriuresis
	↑BP, glucose intolerance, atherosclerosis → MI, stroke
AT-2	Fetus - ?Antigrowth, ?Apoptosis
	Located on adrenal medulla, uterus, ovaries, vascular endothelium
	Cardiac - ?vasodilatory, ?protective
AT-4	?Antifibrinolytic/prothrombotic

(BP: blood pressure; MI: myocardial infarction)

ALDOSTERONE (TABLE 3)

TABLE 3: Aldosterone.[4]

Aldosterone	Stimulates mineralocorticoid receptors in the collecting duct and heart
	Cardiac and renal fibrosis
	Sympathetic over activity in the brainstem

ANGIOTENSIN-CONVERTING ENZYME INHIBITORS

Angiotensin-converting enzyme inhibitors act on the RAAS system, inhibiting the formation of angiotensin II. They cause efferent arteriolar vasodilatation, reducing intraglomerular pressure, and causing effective BP reduction. They are used in mild-to-moderate hypertension as monotherapy or in combination with other classes of drugs. It is beneficial in type 1 diabetics, diabetic nephropathy, and nondiabetic renal disease. In diabetic hypertensive patients with proteinuria and nephropathy, it retards progressive glomerulosclerosis and reduces the progression to renal failure.

Captopril was the first drug in the class. However, because of its side effects, it is rarely used nowadays. The benefits of ACE inhibitors are a group benefit. Enalapril, ramipril, and perindopril have multiple trials with mortality benefit supporting its use. ACE inhibitors are beneficial in postinfarct left ventricular (LV) dysfunction, postinfarct LV remodeling, and heart failure with left ventricular ejection fraction (LVEF) ≤40%. Meta-analysis shows reduction in stroke, coronary artery disease, heart failure, major cardiovascular events, and death.

It is important to monitor renal function and serum K after 1 week of initiation.

PHARMACOLOGIC CHARACTERISTICS OF ANGIOTENSIN-CONVERTING ENZYME INHIBITORS[1] (TABLE 4)

TABLE 4: Pharmacologic characteristics of angiotensin-converting enzyme inhibitors.

Drug	T1/2	Dose (mg/day)	Frequency
Captopril	4–6 hours	25–150 mg	BID
Enalapril (enalaprilat)	6–11 hours	2.5–40 mg	BID
Perindopril (perindoprilat)	3–10 hours	4–16 mg	OD
Ramipril (ramiprilat)	13–17 hours	2.5–20 mg	OD
Trandolapril (trandolaprilat)	10 hours	0.5–8 mg	BID
Lisinopril (water soluble)	7–12 hours	5–80 mg	OD, BID

SIDE EFFECTS OF ANGIOTENSIN-CONVERTING ENZYME INHIBITORS (BOX 1)

Box 1: Side effects of angiotensin-converting enzyme inhibitors.[1]

- Dry cough (5–15%)—due to increased formation of bradykinin
- Orthostatic hypotension
- Hyponatremia, hyperkalemia, and renal failure
- Immune based (taste disturbance, skin rashes, neutropenia)—captopril
- Angioedema

CONTRAINDICATIONS OF ANGIOTENSIN-CONVERTING ENZYME INHIBITORS (BOX 2)

Box 2: Contraindications of angiotensin-converting enzyme inhibitors.[1]

- Bilateral renal artery stenosis
- Pregnancy
- Known hypersensitivity
- Hyperkalemia
- Renal failure (S. creatinine >2.5–3 mg/dL)
- Hypotension
- Severe aortic stenosis, hypertrophic obstructive cardiomyopathy

ANGIOTENSIN RECEPTOR BLOCKERS (TABLE 5)

Angiotensin receptor blockers act on AT1 receptors. Most ARB are metabolized by the liver and excreted in bile or kidneys. Its side effect profile is similar to ACE inhibitors (except dry cough and angioedema). It is very well-tolerated for hypertension because of fewer incidences of dry cough and angioedema. It is advisable to monitor estimated glomerular filtration rate (eGFR) and serum potassium after 1 week of drug initiation and dose change. Dose reduction is required in volume depleted patients. The contraindications are same as ACE inhibitors. ARBs are equally efficacious as ACE inhibitors in reducing cardiovascular (CV) events. The antihypertensive effect begins in 1 week with a peak at 3–6 weeks. For optimum effect, add a diuretic instead of increasing the dose.

There are multiple trials of candesartan, valsartan, telmisartan, and losartan with benefits in patients with postmyocardial infarction (MI) LV dysfunction, heart failure with LVEF ≤40%, diabetic nephropathy, proteinuria of nondiabetic renal disease, and prevention of CV complications. In most

TABLE 5: Angiotensin receptor blockers.[5]

Drug	T1/2	Dose (mg/day)	Frequency
Candesartan	9 hours	8–32 mg	OD, BID
Irbesartan	11–15 hours	75–300 mg	OD
Losartan	6–9 hours	25–100 mg	BID
Telmisartan	24 hours	10–80 mg	OD
Valsartan	6 hours	80–320 mg	OD
Olmesartan	13 hours	5–40 mg	OD
Eprosartan	5–9 hours	400–800 mg	OD, BID
Azilsartan	11 hours	40–80 mg	OD
Fimasartan	9–16 hours	60–120 mg	OD

of the conditions, ARBs are equivalent to ACE inhibitors and can be used interchangeably. However, since ACE inhibitors have more evidence than ARBs in heart failure and post-MI LV dysfunction, ARBs are used only when there is ACE inhibitors intolerance.

Theoretically combination of ACE inhibitor + ARB causes more complete RAAS inhibition with benefits in heart failure, proteinuria of chronic renal disease, and CV protection. However, there is no added mortality benefit, but increased risk of hypotension, renal failure, and dangerous hyperkalemia. Hence, the combination is banned.

MINERALOCORTICOID RECEPTOR ANTAGONISTS

Spironolactone and eplerenone are indicated as add-on agent in resistant hypertension when patient is already on ACE inhibitor/ARB + calcium channel blocker (CCB) + thiazide diuretic. They also have mortality benefit in heart failure with LVEF ≤40% and post-MI LV dysfunction. They are also indicated in primary aldosteronism.

Dosage
- Spironolactone 12.5–100 mg once/twice a day
- Eplerenone 25–100 mg once/twice a day

Side Effects
Spironolactone has a greater risk of gynecomastia and impotence as compared to eplerenone.

Caution
It should be avoided in renal failure and hyperkalemia. It should be used with caution in patients with type 2 diabetes with renal insufficiency and other drugs which cause hyperkalemia. It is advisable to monitor serum creatinine and serum K levels.

DIRECT RENIN INHIBITION

Let us have a look at the RAAS system. Diuretics, ACE inhibitors, and ARBs increase renin and plasma renin activity. Renin causes increase in BP and renal dysfunction. Theoretically, addition of renin inhibitor, aliskiren, should cause more complete RAAS inhibition and effective control of BP. However, studies were halted prematurely as there was an increased risk of stroke, renal failure, hyperkalemia, and hypotension when aliskiren 300 mg was added to ACE inhibitor or ARB. It is contraindicated in bilateral renal artery stenosis and pregnancy.

Dose
Aliskiren 75–300 mg OD.

SUMMARY

- ACE inhibitors/ARB can be used in combination with other classes of drugs, except renin inhibitors.
- ACE inhibitors are more protective in patients of diabetes, proteinuria, and chronic kidney disease (CKD) and used as first line.
- ACE inhibitors and ARBs are first-line agent for diabetic and nondiabetic proteinuric CKD.
- ACE inhibitors and ARBs are drugs of choice for left ventricular hypertrophy, heart failure, and post-MI LV dysfunction. ARBs are used only in ACE intolerant patients.
- They are less effective than CCBs in lowering BP in black and older patients with low renin activity. It is better to use them in combination with CCBs in such cases.
- ARBs have similar benefits as ACE inhibitors except dry cough and angioedema.
- Direct renin inhibitor, aliskiren, is not advisable. Combination of any of the RAAS inhibitors can cause hypotension, renal failure, and hyperkalemia and is contraindicated.
- All RAAS inhibitors are contraindicated in pregnancy.
- Monitoring of renal function and potassium is recommended.

MULTIPLE CHOICE QUESTIONS

1. The recommended RAAS inhibitor combination is:
   A. ACE inhibitor + ARB
   B. ARB + direct renin inhibitor
   C. ACE inhibitor + ARB + direct rennin inhibitor
   D. None of the above

2. In patients of diabetes, the recommended first-line antihypertensive is:
   A. ACE inhibitor
   B. ARB
   C. CCB
   D. Any of the above

3. The following is the side effect of ARB, *except*:
   A. Angioedema
   B. Hyperkalemia
   C. Renal failure
   D. Hyponatremia

4. The following is a contraindication of ACE inhibitors, *except*:
   A. Hyperkalemia
   B. Hypotension
   C. Renal failure
   D. Heart failure with reduced ejection fraction

5. The following investigations are to be done after prescribing mineralocorticoid receptor antagonist (MRA), *except*:
   A. Serum creatinine
   B. Serum electrolytes
   C. Urine microalbumin
   D. Creatinine phosphokinase

Answers

1—D   2—D   3—A   4—D   5—D

REFERENCES

1. Goyal A, Cusick AS, Thielemier B. ACE Inhibitors. In: StatPearls. Treasure Island (FL): StatPearls Publishing; 2022.
2. Herman LL, Padala SA, Ahmed I, Bashir K. Angiotensin Converting Enzyme Inhibitors (ACEI). In: StatPearls. Treasure Island (FL): StatPearls Publishing; 2022.
3. Singh KD, Karnik SS. Angiotensin receptors: Structure, function, signaling and clinical applications. J Cell Signal. 2016;1(2):111.
4. Guichard JL, Clark D 3rd, Calhoun DA, Ahmed MI. Aldosterone receptor antagonists: current perspectives and therapies. Vasc Health Risk Manag. 2013;9:321-31.
5. Hill RD, Vaidya PN. Angiotensin II Receptor Blockers (ARB). In: StatPearls. Treasure Island (FL): StatPearls Publishing; 2022.

SUGGESTED READINGS

1. Chen R, Suchard MA, Krumholz HM, Schuemie MJ, Shea S, Duke J, et al. Comparative first-line effectiveness and safety of ACE (angiotensin-converting enzyme) inhibitors and angiotensin receptor blockers: A multinational cohort study. Hypertension. 2021;78(3):591-603.
2. Materson BJ. Monotherapy of hypertension with angiotensin-converting enzyme inhibitors. Am J Med. 1984;77(4A):128-34.
3. Frank GJ. The safety of ACE inhibitors for the treatment of hypertension and congestive heart failure. Cardiology. 1989;76 (Suppl 2):56-67.
4. Li EC, Heran BS, Wright JM. Angiotensin converting enzyme (ACE) inhibitors versus angiotensin receptor blockers for primary hypertension. Cochrane Database Syst Rev. 2014;2014(8):CD009096.
5. Wang GM, Li LJ, Tang WL, Wright JM. Renin inhibitors versus angiotensin converting enzyme (ACE) inhibitors for primary hypertension. Cochrane Database Syst Rev. 2020;10(10):CD012569.
6. Azizi M, Webb R, Nussberger J, Hollenberg NK. Renin inhibition with aliskiren: where are we now, and where are we going. J Hypertens. 2006;24(2):243-6.
7. Shafiq MM, Menon DV, Victor RG. Oral direct renin inhibition: Premise, promise, and potential limitations of a new class of antihypertensive drug. Am J Med. 2008;121(4):265-71.

4.2 Calcium Channel Blockers

Ruchit Shah

INTRODUCTION

Calcium (Ca) enters through the L type and T type calcium channels. Calcium channel blockers (CCBs) inhibit the Ca entry in smooth muscles and myocardium. CCBs cause peripheral vasodilatation, reduction of peripheral vascular resistance, and negative inotropy. They are chemically dihydropyridines (DHP) and nondihydropyridines (non-DHP) **(Table 1)**.

TABLE 1: Calcium channel blockers: Dihydropyridines (DHP) and nondihydropyridines (non–DHP).[1-3]

DHP	Non-DHP
• Nifedipine (short-acting) • Nifedipine (N) (long-acting) • Amlodipine (A) (long-acting)	• Verapamil (V) (IV, oral, slow release) • Diltiazem (D) (IV, oral, slow release)
Acts on alpha-1 subunit (N site)	Acts on two different sites of alpha-1 subunit
Acts predominantly on vascular smooth muscle	Acts predominantly on AV node and SA node
Used for angina (effort, vasospastic), hypertension, Raynaud's phenomenon	Used for angina (vasospastic, effort, unstable), hypertension, supraventricular arrhythmias, rate control in atrial fibrillation/ flutter
• *Side effects:* Headache, bilateral ankle edema • Dizziness, flushing (A)	• *Side effects:* Vasodilatation → headache, facial flushing, dizziness, constipation, AV blocks • Ankle edema (D)
Contraindication: Unstable angina, post-MI, heart failure, severe aortic stenosis, obstructive cardiomyopathy, pre-existing ↓BP	Contraindicated in bradyarrhythmias, heart failure, post-MI, LVEF ≤ 40%, ventricular arrhythmias

Continued

Continued

DHP	Non-DHP
Drug interactions: Nifedipine causes ↑ LV depression with beta blockade. Avoid in unstable angina without beta blockade. N and A act via CYP3A4 and interact with simvastatin (limit dose to <20 mg). Liver disease → ↑ blood levels of N and A	• *Drug interactions:* V levels ↑in liver or renal disease, digoxin level ↑ (V), statin level ↑ (V, D) • V and D inhibit CYP3A • It is advisable to avoid intravenous (IV) preparations with beta blockers
(A: amlodipine; AV: atrioventricular; CYP: cytochrome P; D: diltiazem; DHP: dihydropyridines; LVEF: left ventricular ejection fraction; LV: left ventricle; MI: myocardial infarction; N: nifedipine; SA: sinoatrial node; V: verapamil)	

PHARMACOLOGICAL PROPERTIES OF CALCIUM CHANNEL BLOCKERS (TABLE 2)

TABLE 2: Pharmacological properties of calcium channel blockers.[3-8]

Drug	T1/2	Dose (mg/day)	Frequency
Verapamil	3–7 hours	120–480 mg	OD, BID, TID
Diltiazem	3–4.5 hours	120–360 mg	OD, BID, QID
Nifedipine (long-acting)	6–12 hours	30–120 mg	OD
Amlodipine	35–48 hours	2.5–10 mg	OD
S-amlodipine		2.5–10 mg	OD
Cilnidipine	20 minutes	5–10 mg	OD
Benidipine	1 hour	4–8 mg	OD
Efonidipine	4 hours	20–40 mg	OD
Felodipine	25 hours	2.5–20 mg	OD, BID

- Verapamil is excreted by the kidney (75%) and the liver (25%).
- Diltiazem is excreted by the kidney (35%) and the liver (65%).
- *Nifedipine (short-acting)*: It is indicated in attacks of vasospastic angina or Raynaud's phenomenon. It causes rapid arteriolar vasodilatation, hypotension, and may precipitate ischemia. Hence, it is contraindicated in unstable angina.
- *Nifedipine (long-acting)*: It is excreted by the kidneys. It is used in effort angina, Prinzmetal vasospastic angina, hypertension (HTN), and Raynaud's phenomenon. It can be used in HTN patients having angina in combination with a beta blocker. It should not be used in unstable angina.
- Amlodipine is the most commonly used drug. It has a slow onset and long duration of action and is given in once-a-day dose. It has well-tolerated side effects. Dose needs to be reduced in older individuals. Amlodipine can be given as a monotherapy or combination with angiotensin-converting enzyme (ACE) inhibitors/angiotensin receptor blocker (ARB)/diuretics for management of HTN. It has many large trials with proven outcome

benefits to its credit. It can also be used for effort angina. Though heart failure is a contraindication to the use of CCB, amlodipine can be used with caution in controlled heart failure.
- There are a few studies suggesting more renoprotective effects with cilnidipine. A few studies have shown lacidipine to be beneficial in carotid atherosclerosis with lesser incidence of new metabolic syndrome. Lacidipine also has lesser ankle edema than amlodipine. Benidipine has been observed to have beneficial effects on cardiac remodeling.

Calcium channel blockers are commonly used for HTN as a first-line agent. CCBs achieve marked reduction of blood pressure (BP), cardiovascular (CV) outcomes, stroke, carotid atherosclerosis, and mortality benefit. CCBs have lesser incidence of stroke and higher incidence of heart failure. They are as effective as ACE inhibitors/ARBs/diuretics.

SUMMARY

- DHP CCBs (e.g., amlodipine) are used as first-line agents for control of HTN. They can be used alone or in combination with other classes of drugs.
- CCBs have many advantages compared to other classes of drugs. They do not have metabolic side effects and do not require monitoring of electrolytes and renal parameters. They are efficacious, relatively safe, and well-tolerated.
- Of the CCBs, amlodipine is most widely studied and used. CCBs are more effective in stroke.

MULTIPLE CHOICE QUESTIONS

1. The preferred CCB in HTN is:
   A. Nifedipine
   B. Amlodipine
   C. Verapamil
   D. Diltiazem

2. Pedal edema of amlodipine can be treated by:
   A. Fluid restriction
   B. Diuretic
   C. ACE inhibitors
   D. Change drug to cilnidipine

3. Which of the following combination can dangerous bradycardia?
   A. Verapamil + beta blocker
   B. Amlodipine + beta blocker
   C. Beta blocker + diuretic
   D. Nifedipine + diltiazem

4. Which of the following is a contraindication for nifedipine?
   A. Prinzmetal vasospastic angina
   B. Unstable angina
   C. Effort angina
   D. Stable angina

5. Which of the following can be used with caution in heart failure?
   A. Nifedipine
   B. Amlodipine
   C. Verapamil
   D. Diltiazem

Answers

1—B 2—C 3—A 4—B 5—B

REFERENCES

1. Frishman WH. Calcium channel blockers: Differences between subclasses. Am J Cardiovasc Drugs. 2007;7 (Suppl 1):17-23.
2. Katz AM. Pharmacology and mechanisms of action of calcium-channel blockers. J Clin Hypertens. 1986;2(3 Suppl):28S-37S.
3. McKeever RG, Hamilton RJ. Calcium channel blockers. In: StatPearls. Treasure Island (FL): StatPearls Publishing; 2022.
4. McDonagh MS, Eden KB, Peterson K. Drug class review: Calcium channel blockers: Final Report. Portland (OR): Oregon Health & Science University; 2005.
5. Rameis H. Grundlagen der Pharmakokinetik und Pharmakodynamik von Kalziumantagonisten [Principles of the pharmacokinetics and pharmacodynamics of calcium antagonists]. Wien Med Wochenschr. 1993;143(19-20):490-500.
6. Scholz H. Pharmacological aspects of calcium channel blockers. Cardiovasc Drugs Ther. 1997;10 (Suppl 3):869-72.
7. Katz AM, Hager WD, Messineo FC, Pappano AJ. Cellular actions and pharmacology of the calcium channel blocking drugs. Am J Med. 1984;77(2B):2-10.
8. Bulsara KG, Cassagnol M. Amlodipine. In: StatPearls. Treasure Island (FL): StatPearls Publishing; 2022.

SUGGESTED READINGS

1. Neutel JM. Complementary mechanisms of angiotensin receptor blockers and calcium channel blockers in managing hypertension. Postgrad Med. 2009;121(2):40-8.
2. Tiwaskar M, Langote A, Kashyap R, Toppo A. Amlodipine in the era of new generation calcium channel blockers. J Assoc Physicians India. 2018;66(3):64-9.
3. Tran KC, Leung AA, Tang KL, Quan H, Khan NA. Efficacy of calcium channel blockers on major cardiovascular outcomes for the treatment of hypertension in Asian populations: A meta-analysis. Can J Cardiol. 2017;33(5):635-43.
4. Pontremoli R, Leoncini G, Parodi A. Use of nifedipine in the treatment of hypertension. Expert Rev Cardiovasc Ther. 2005;3(1):43-50.
5. Sierra C, Coca A. The ACTION study: Nifedipine in patients with symptomatic stable angina and hypertension. Expert Rev Cardiovasc Ther. 2008;6(8):1055-62.

4.3 Diuretics

Amjad Khan

INTRODUCTION

There are various groups of diuretics acting on different sites of the nephron causing sequential nephron blockade. In hypertension, diuretics cause natriuresis, volume depletion, and vasodilatation **(Fig. 1)**.

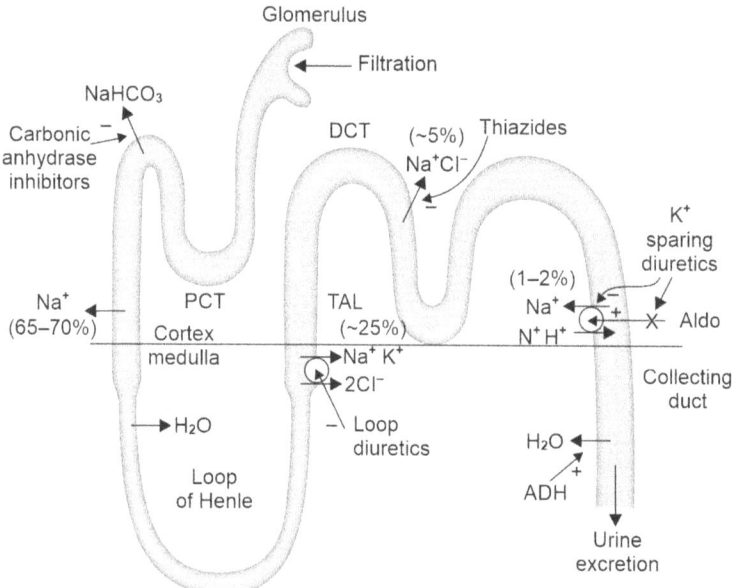

FIG. 1: Nephron showing different sites of action of various diuretics.
(ADH: antidiuretic hormone; DCT: distal convoluted tubule; PCT: proximal convoluted tubule; TAL: thick ascending limb of loop of Henle)

CLASSES OF DIURETICS (TABLE 1)

TABLE 1: Classes of diuretics.[1-8]

Thiazides/ thiazide-like	Loop diuretics	K-sparing diuretics	Aquaretics
• Hydrochlorothiazide • Chlorthalidone • Indapamide • Metolazone	• Furosemide • Torsemide • Bumetanide	• Amiloride (A) • Triamterene (T) • Spironolactone (S) • Eplerenone (E)	• Tolvaptan • Conivaptan • Satavaptan • Lixivaptan
Inhibit Na^+/Cl^- cotransporter in distal convoluted tubule (DCT)	• Inhibits $Na^+/K^+/2Cl^-$ cotransporter in ascending limb of loop of Henle • Venodilatation, diuresis → preload reduction	• A acts on renal epithelial Na channel and T inhibits Na-proton exchanger in DCT and collecting tubules • S and E are mineralocorticoid receptor antagonists	Inhibits aquaporin-2 (AVP-2 receptor antagonists)—located on collecting ducts → It causes free water clearance, decreased urine osmolality, and ↑serum Na
Use: Hypertension, heart failure	*Use*: Heart failure, hypertensive crisis, and hypertension	*Use*: Resistant hypertension, primary aldosteronism, and heart failure	*Use*: heart failure with hyponatremia
S/E: ↓K→ arrhythmias, ↓Na, ↓Mg, hyperglycemia, hyperuricemia, prerenal azotemia, lipid profile derangements, nausea, dizziness, and impotence	S/E: ↓K → arrhythmias, hypovolemia → azotemia, hyperglycemia, lipid profile derangements, and ototoxicity	S/E: ↑K	S/E: ↓BP, thirst
Avoid in pregnancy and severe renal failure	Avoid in pregnancy, lactation, combination with nephrotoxic drugs and NSAIDs	Avoid in acute/chronic renal failure, ↑K	

(A: amiloride; AVP: arginine vasopressin; Cl: chloride; DCT: distal convoluted tubule; E: eplerenone; K: potassium; Mg: magnesium; Na: sodium; NSAIDs: nonsteroidal anti-inflammatory drugs; PCT: proximal convoluted tubule; S: spironolactone; T: triamterene)

PHARMACOLOGICAL CHARACTERISTICS OF DIURETICS (TABLE 2)

Most of the diuretics are excreted by the kidneys. Tolvaptan is excreted by the liver.

Thiazides maximal response is achieved at a low dose (low-ceiling diuretics). Low-dose thiazide diuretics are most widely used for hypertension alone or in combination with other classes of drugs. High-dose thiazides can be used in heart failure in combination with loop diuretics. They do not act in presence of renal failure.

There are no comparison studies between different thiazides. Chlorthalidone is longer acting than hydrochlorothiazide and achieves a sustained reduction in BP; hence, it is a preferred drug. Chlorthalidone and indapamide have multiple trials to support their use in hypertension. Low-dose thiazide diuretics reduce stroke, coronary artery disease with mortality benefit in old adults with mild-to-moderate hypertension.

Metolazone is a powerful thiazide diuretic. It can be used in combination with loop diuretics in heart failure. It acts even in presence of renal failure.

Most of the side effects of thiazides can be overcome by using low doses, in combination with angiotensin-converting enzyme (ACE) inhibitors/angiotensin receptor blocker (ARB) for hypertension and adding a K-sparing diuretic. Monitoring of renal function and electrolytes is advisable.

TABLE 2: Pharmacological characteristics of diuretics.[6-9]

Drug	Duration of action	Dose (mg/day)	Frequency
Thiazide/thiazide-like			
Hydrochlorothiazide	16–24 hours	6.25–100 mg	OD
Chlorthalidone	40–60 hours	6.25–50 mg	OD
Metolazone	24 hours	2.5–5 mg	OD
Indapamide	24 hours	0.625–2.5 mg	OD
Loop diuretics			
Furosemide	4–5 hours	20–160 mg oral/IV	BID
Torsemide	6–8 hours	2.5–200 mg oral/IV	OD, BID
Bumetanide	4–5 hours	0.5–2 mg oral/IV	BID
K-sparing diuretics			
Amiloride	6–24 hours	5–20 mg	OD
Triamterene	8–12 hours	25–100 mg	OD
Spironolactone	3–5 days	12.5–100 mg	OD, BID
Eplerenone	24 hours	25–100 mg	OD, BID
Aquaretics			
Tolvaptan	12 hours	30–90 mg	OD, BID
(IV: intravenous)			

Loop diuretics have a dose-dependent increase in their effect (high-ceiling diuretics). They are used intravenously in heart failure. Combination of two or more diuretics acting at different sites of the nephron is used to achieve sequential nephron blockade. This helps to achieve better diuresis and limit the metabolic side effects. They can also be used in presence of renal insufficiency and hypertensive emergencies. Higher doses of loop diuretics cause metabolic derangements, hence renal function, and electrolytes should be monitored.

Potassium-sparing diuretics can be used in combination with other diuretics to reduce the risk of hypokalemia and dangerous ventricular arrhythmias. They are also useful in resistant hypertension and primary aldosteronism.

Aquaretics: Arginine vasopressin receptor (AVP-2) antagonists: They are mainly used in heart failure with hyponatremia. *They have limited role in hypertension.*

Carbonic anhydrase inhibitors, e.g., acetazolamide—it acts on the proximal convoluted tubule to decrease secretion of H^+ ions and loss of HCO_3^- and Na^+ ions. It is used in glaucoma and altitude sickness.

Mannitol—it acts on the proximal convoluted tubule. *It has no role in hypertension.*

SUMMARY

- Thiazide diuretics (chlorthalidone, indapamide > hydrochlorothiazide) are the first-line agents in hypertension treatment. They are best used in low dose to avert the side effects. Combining it with an ACE inhibitor/ARB or other classes of drugs helps to achieve better BP control.
- Loop diuretics are primarily indicated for treatment of symptomatic heart failure.
- Potassium-sparing diuretics are used for resistant hypertension. They can be used as add-on therapy for sequential nephron blockade and preventing hypokalemia-induced dangerous ventricular arrhythmias.
- All diuretics cause volume contraction, azotemia, and electrolyte disturbances. It is advisable to monitor renal function and electrolytes.

MULTIPLE CHOICE QUESTIONS

1. In patient with normal eGFR, which is the preferred diuretic for management of hypertension?
    A. Loop diuretic
    B. Thiazide diuretic
    C. Potassium-sparing diuretic
    D. Osmotic diuretic

2. In patient with CKD stages 3–5, which is the preferred diuretic for management of hypertension?
    A. Loop diuretic
    B. Thiazide diuretic

C. Potassium-sparing diuretic
D. Osmotic diuretic

3. Thiazide-like diuretic which retains its activity at lower eGFR:
   A. Metolazone
   B. Hydrochlorothiazide
   C. Chlorthalidone
   D. Indapamide

4. In patient with heart failure, which is the preferred diuretic for management of hyponatremia?
   A. Metolazone
   B. Eplerenone (E)
   C. Tolvaptan
   D. Bumetanide

5. Which of the following is not a side effect of thiazide/thiazide-like diuretic?
   A. Hyperglycemia
   B. Hyperuricemia
   C. Hyperkalemia
   D. Hyponatremia

Answers

1—B   2—A   3—A   4—C   5—C

REFERENCES

1. Roush GC, Sica DA. Diuretics for hypertension: A review and update. Am J Hypertens. 2016;29(10):1130-7.
2. Shah S, Khatri I, Freis ED. Mechanism of antihypertensive effect of thiazide diuretics. Am Heart J. 1978;95(5):611-8.
3. Mishra S. Diuretics in primary hypertension: Reloaded. Indian Heart J. 2016;68(5):720-3.
4. O'Donovan RA, Muhammedi M, Puschett JB. Diuretics in the therapy of hypertension: current status. Am J Med Sci. 1992;304(5):312-8.
5. Blowey DL. Diuretics in the treatment of hypertension. Pediatr Nephrol. 2016;31(12):2223-33.
6. Huxel C, Raja A, Ollivierre-Lawrence MD. Loop diuretics. In: StatPearls. Treasure Island (FL): StatPearls Publishing; 2021.
7. Akbari P, Khorasani-Zadeh A. Thiazide diuretics. In: StatPearls. Treasure Island (FL): StatPearls Publishing; 2022.
8. Arumugham VB, Shahin MH. Therapeutic uses of diuretic agents. In: StatPearls. StatPearls Publishing; Treasure Island (FL): 2022.
9. James PA, Oparil S, Carter BL, Cushman WC, Dennison-Himmelfarb C, Handler J, et al. 2014 evidence-based guideline for the management of high blood pressure in adults: report from the panel members appointed to the Eighth Joint National Committee (JNC 8). JAMA. 2014;311(5):507-20.

SUGGESTED READINGS

1. Antonietta CM, Calvi E, Faggiano A, Maffeis C, Bosisio M, De Stefano M, et al. Impact of loop diuretic on outcomes in patients with heart failure and reduced ejection fraction. Curr Heart Fail Rep. 2022;19(1):15-25.
2. Wargo KA, Banta WM. A comprehensive review of the loop diuretics: should furosemide be first line? Ann Pharmacother. 2009;43(11):1836-47.
3. Tamargo J, Segura J, Ruilope LM. Diuretics in the treatment of hypertension. Part 1: thiazide and thiazide-like diuretics. Expert Opin Pharmacother. 2014;15(4):527-47.
4. Malha L, Mann SJ. Loop diuretics in the treatment of hypertension. Curr Hypertens Rep. 2016;18(4):27.

4.4 Beta-blockers

Ruchit Shah

MECHANISM

- Beta-1 receptors—located on cardiac sarcolemma
- Beta-2 receptors—located on bronchial and vascular smooth muscle
- Beta-3 receptors—located on endothelium

EFFECTS OF BETA-BLOCKERS

- Negative chronotropic effect (sinus node pacemaker current is reduced)
- Negative dromotropic effect (rate of cardiac contraction is decreased)
- Negative inotropic effect (reduced myocardial contraction)
- Antiarrhythmic effect
- Anti-ischemic effect—decreased myocardial oxygen demand (decreased heart rate, decreased afterload, decreased contractility, decreased O_2 wastage, increased diastolic perfusion, and less exercise-induced vasoconstriction)
- Antihypertensive effect—decreased cardiac output (beta 1), renin release (beta 1), and norepinephrine release (beta 2)

PHARMACOLOGIC PROPERTIES OF BETA-BLOCKERS (TABLE 1)

TABLE 1: Pharmacologic properties of beta-blockers.[1-4]

Drug	T1/2	Dose (mg/day)	Frequency
Noncardioselective			
Propranolol	1–6 hours	40–180 mg	BID
Carteolol	5–6 hours	2.5–10 mg	OD
Nadolol	20–24 hours	20–320 mg	OD
Sotalol	7–18 hours	80–320 mg	BID
Timolol	4–5 hours	20–60 mg	BID
Cardioselective			
Acebutolol	8–13 hours	200–800 mg	BID
Atenolol	6–7 hours	25–100 mg	OD

Continued

Continued

Drug	T1/2	Dose (mg/day)	Frequency
Bisoprolol	9–12 hours	2.5–20 mg	OD
Metoprolol XL	3–7 hours	50–200 mg	OD/BID
Vasodilatory, nonselective (alpha + beta-blockers)			
Labetalol	6–8 hours	200–2,400 mg	QID
Carvedilol	6 hours	6.25–50 mg	BID
Carvedilol CR		10–40 mg	OD
Vasodilatory, selective			
Nebivolol	10 hours	5–40 mg	OD

- Beta-blockers are weak antihypertensives and *are not used as first line agents*.
- They reduce the central aortic pressure less than the brachial pressure.
- They are used in young hypertensives, angina, and postmyocardial infarction (MI) patients with hypertension in combination with other classes of drugs. The Cochrane review summarizes that other classes of antihypertensive drugs are better than beta-blockers in preventing death, stroke, and heart attacks.
- Beta-blockers have an undisputed mortality benefit in patients of heart failure, arrhythmias, and post-MI. Bisoprolol, metoprolol, and carvedilol have trials with proven mortality benefit in patients with heart failure.
- They are also used for hypertrophic obstructive cardiomyopathy, mitral stenosis, mitral valve prolapse, dissecting aneurysm, Marfan syndrome, tetralogy of Fallot, thyrotoxicosis, anxiety, glaucoma, migraine, and esophageal varices.
- Chronic beta-blockade therapy increases beta receptor density. Abrupt withdrawal may precipitate angina or MI. If beta-blockers need to be stopped, it must be done gradually with slow tapering of the drug.
- There is increased risk of diabetes when used in combination with a diuretic. Fatigability leads to drug discontinuation. Weight gain, bronchospasm, and conduction disturbances are other limiting side effects.
- Esmolol is an ultra short-acting beta-blocker with t1/2 of 9 minutes. It is given intravenously in patients with emergency hypertension, perioperative hypertension, supraventricular tachycardia, acute coronary syndrome with heart failure requiring short-acting beta-blockade.
- Nebivolol causes nitric oxide (NO)-mediated vasodilatation. It has favorable effects on central BP, aortic stiffness, and endothelial dysfunction. It does not cause new-onset diabetes mellitus and lesser chances of sexual dysfunction.
- Cardioselective agents (beta 1 selective) such as metoprolol, bisoprolol, and atenolol can be used in patients with chronic lung disease and insulin-dependent diabetes mellitus. It has less bronchospasm and lesser metabolic effects. Bisoprolol is the most cardioselective among all.

SIDE EFFECTS (BOX 1)

Box 1: Side effects.[1]

- Bronchospasm
- Cold extremities, worsening of claudication
- Bradycardia, heart block
- Worsening of heart failure
- Insomnia, depression
- Fatigue
- Weight gain
- Worsening of diabetes, ↑triglyceride, ↓HDL
- Erectile dysfunction

(HDL: high-density lipoprotein)

CONTRAINDICATIONS (TABLE 2)

TABLE 2: Contraindications.[1]

Absolute	Relative
Cardiac: Severe bradycardia, high grade AV block, cardiogenic shock, untreated heart failure	*Cardiac*: Prinzmetal angina—avoid sudden withdrawal
Respiratory: Severe asthma and bronchospasm	*Respiratory*: Mild asthma—use cardioselective agents at lower dose
Central nervous system: Severe depression	*Central nervous system*: Vivid dreams, visual hallucinations
Peripheral vascular disease: Severe peripheral vascular disease, gangrene, skin necrosis, and rest claudication	*Peripheral vascular disease*: Raynaud phenomenon—avoid nonselective agents such as propranolol, prefer vasodilatory agents
	Diabetes, metabolic syndrome, and dyslipidemia
	Renal failure: Avoid drugs excreted by the kidney. Dose adjustment may be required
	Liver failure: Avoid drugs with hepatic excretion
(AV: arteriovenous)	

SUMMARY

- Beta-blockers are not indicated as a first-line agent for treatment of hypertension. They can be used in combination with other classes of drugs for more compelling indications. One needs to be cautious about the side effects and contraindications.
- Metoprolol, carvedilol, and bisoprolol have mortality benefit in patients with heart failure and post-MI.
- Cardioselective beta-blockers may be given in patients with mild-to-moderate bronchospasm.

CHAPTER 4 Drug Therapy

MULTIPLE CHOICE QUESTIONS

1. Which is the most cardioselective beta-blocker?
   A. Carvedilol
   B. Metoprolol
   C. Nebivolol
   D. Bisoprolol

2. Beta-blockers may be used with caution in all, *except*:
   A. Mild bronchial asthma
   B. Chronic heart failure
   C. First degree arteriovenous (AV) block
   D. Peripheral vascular disease

3. The preferred beta-blocker in old age individuals >65 years is:
   A. Nebivolol
   B. Propranolol
   C. Esmolol
   D. Timolol

4. Beta-blockers have relative contraindication in the following, *except*:
   A. Hyperthyroidism
   B. Diabetes mellitus
   C. Metabolic syndrome
   D. Dyslipidemia

5. Which of these is a false statement?
   A. Beta-blocker shows negative inotropic effect
   B. Beta-blockers have antiarrhythmic effect
   C. Beta-blocker shows negative dromotropic effect
   D. Beta-blocker shows positive chronotropic effect

Answers

1—D   2—B   3—A   4—A   5—D

REFERENCES

1. Farzam K, Jan A. Beta blockers. In: StatPearls. Treasure Island (FL): StatPearls Publishing; 2022.
2. do Vale GT, Ceron CS, Gonzaga NA, Simplicio JA, Padovan JC. Three generations of β-blockers: History, class differences and clinical applicability. Curr Hypertens Rev. 2019;15(1):22-31.
3. Gorre F, Vandekerckhove H. Beta-blockers: focus on mechanism of action. Which beta-blocker, when and why? Acta Cardiol. 2010;65(5):565-70.
4. Wiysonge CS, Bradley HA, Volmink J, Mayosi BM, Opie LH. Beta-blockers for hypertension. Cochrane Database Syst Rev. 2017;1(1):CD002003.

SUGGESTED READINGS

1. Oliver E, Mayor F Jr, D'Ocon P. Beta-blockers: Historical perspective and mechanisms of action. Rev Esp Cardiol (Engl Ed). 2019;72(10):853-62.
2. Weir MR. Beta-blockers in the treatment of hypertension: are there clinically relevant differences? Postgrad Med. 2009;121(3):90-8.
3. Weber MA. The role of the new beta-blockers in treating cardiovascular disease. Am J Hypertens. 2005;18(12 Pt 2):169S-76S.
4. Ogrodowczyk M, Dettlaff K, Jelinska A. Beta-blockers: Current state of knowledge and perspectives. Mini Rev Med Chem. 2016;16(1):40-54.

4.5 Other Drugs

Sudhiranjan Dash Choudhury, Ruchit Shah

INTRODUCTION

Apart from the main classes of drugs being used as first-line therapy for hypertension, there are other drugs which can be used as an add-on therapy for specific indications only.

SUMMARY OF OTHER CLASSES OF ANTIHYPERTENSIVES (TABLE 1)

TABLE 1: Other classes of antihypertensives.[1-5]

Alpha-blockers	Central sympatholytics	Vasodilators
Alpha 1 selective blockers: • Prazosin (1–40 mg/day BID, TID) • Terazosin (1–20 mg/day OD) • Doxazosin (1–16 mg/day OD) • Phenoxybenzamine 20–120 mg/day BID	• Clonidine 0.3–1.2 mg/day TID • Alpha methyldopa 250–1,000 mg/day BID • Moxonidine 0.2–0.4 mg/day OD/BID • Guanabenz 2–32 mg/day BID • Guanfacine 1–3 mg at night, • Reserpine 0.05–0.25 mg/day OD	• Hydralazine 25–300 mg/day TID • Minoxidil 2.5–100 mg/day OD/BID
Block sympathetic over activity (norepinephrine release ↓→↓ peripheral vascular resistance → ↓BP)	This causes reduced adrenergic drive to heart and peripheral circulation	Opens vascular ATP sensitive K channels → arterial vasodilatation
Use: Resistant hypertension, benign prostatic hypertrophy, chronic kidney disease, glucose intolerance, and dyslipidemia	*Use*: Alpha methyldopa—hypertension in pregnancy, resistant hypertension Clonidine—resistant hypertension and chronic kidney disease	*Use*: Resistant hypertension and hypertension in pregnancy

Continued

Continued

Alpha-blockers	Central sympatholytics	Vasodilators
S/E: Orthostatic hypotension, drowsiness, diarrhea, and tachycardia. Tolerance occurs due to fluid retention	S/E: Clonidine—postural hypotension, anticholinergic effects, withdrawal related rebound hypertension	S/E: Tachycardia, headache, Na and water retention. Hydralazine can cause lupus. Minoxidil can cause hirsutism and pericarditis
C/I: Heart failure	• C/I: Alpha methyldopa—liver disease • Clonidine—pregnancy, lactation	Use with caution in coronary artery disease
(C/I: contraindications; S/E: side effects)		

ALPHA-BLOCKERS

Alpha 1 selective blockers cause fluid retention and tachyphylaxis leading to heart failure. It is used as add-on therapy in combination with a diuretic for difficult hypertension. It also dilates the urethral muscles, hence preferred in older men with benign hypertrophy of the prostate. Orthostatic hypotension can be dangerous; hence, postural BP must be assessed at every clinic visit.
- Phenoxybenzamine is used preoperatively for pheochromocytoma. Once alpha blockade is achieved, beta-blockers are added to control reflex tachycardia.

CENTRAL SYMPATHOLYTICS

They are used as an add-on therapy of hypertensive urgency, when beta-blockers are contraindicated. Stimulation of postsynaptic alpha 2 and imidazoline receptors in central nervous system causes reduced central sympathetic outflow. Stimulation of presynaptic alpha 2 receptors causes reduced norepinephrine release from peripheral sympathetic nerves. The combination of this leads to reduced adrenergic drive to heart and peripheral circulation.
- Reserpine can be used in a low dose with diuretics.
- Alpha methyldopa acts on central alpha 2 receptors.
- Transdermal clonidine reduces the risk of clonidine rebound.
- Guanfacine can be given once a day at night with less risk of rebound.
- Moxonidine is an imidazoline receptor blocker.

DIRECT VASODILATORS

It causes rapid arteriolar vasodilatation which leads to profound reflex sympathetic activation and tachycardia.

- Hydralazine is used for preeclampsia and difficult hypertension.
- Hydralazine + isosorbide dinitrate is used for heart failure with preserved ejection fraction.
- Minoxidil + beta-blocker + loop diuretic are used in severe hypertension with chronic kidney disease.

SUMMARY

- Alpha-blockers block sympathetic over activity and commonly used for resistant hypertension, BPH, CKD, glucose intolerance and dyslipidemia.
- Central sympatholytics reduce adrenergic drive to heart and peripheral circulation.
- Alphamethyl dopa can be used for gestational hypertension and resistant hypertension.
- Clonididine is contraindicated in pregnancy and lactation.
- Vasodilators open vadcular ATP sensitive K channels and are used for resistant as well as gestational hypertension.

MULTIPLE CHOICE QUESTIONS

1. All of the following cause postural hypotension, *except*:
   A. Moxonidine
   B. Minoxidil
   C. Prazosin
   D. Guanabenz

2. This drug can be given in heart failure:
   A. Terazosin
   B. Alpha methyldopa
   C. Reserpine
   D. Hydralazine

3. Drug which causes lupus-like reaction:
   A. Minoxidil
   B. Phenoxybenzamine
   C. Hydralazine
   D. Phentolamine

4. Which of the following is not a side effect of minoxidil?
   A. Hirsutism
   B. Pericarditis
   C. Headache
   D. Bradycardia

5. Alpha blockers can be used in the following conditions, *except*:
   A. Pheochromocytoma
   B. Heart failure

C. Dyslipidemia
D. Benign hypertrophy of the prostrate

Answers

1—B   2—D   3—C   4—D   5—B

REFERENCES

1. Reddy KS, Prabhakaran D. Combination of alpha-blockers with other antihypertensive drugs. J Assoc Physicians India. 1998;Suppl 1:22-5.
2. Rossitto G, Kamath G, Messerli FH. Should alpha-blockers ever be used as antihypertensive drugs. Cleve Clin J Med. 2010;77(12):884-8.
3. Vongpatanasin W, Kario K, Atlas SA, Victor RG. Central sympatholytic drugs. J Clin Hypertens (Greenwich). 2011;13(9):658-61.
4. Sica DA. Minoxidil: an underused vasodilator for resistant or severe hypertension. J Clin Hypertens (Greenwich). 2004;6(5):283-7.
5. Hariri L, Patel JB. Vasodilators. In: StatPearls. Treasure Island (FL): StatPearls Publishing; 2022.

SUGGESTED READINGS

1. Frishman WH, Kotob F. Alpha-adrenergic blocking drugs in clinical medicine. J Clin Pharmacol. 1999;39(1):7-16.
2. Kaplan SA. Retreatment patterns in alpha-blocker therapy for benign prostatic hyperplasia. J Urol. 2015;193(5):1593-4.
3. Hanna J, Ghazi L, Yamamoto Y, Simonov M, Shah T, Wilson FP, et al. Excessive blood pressure response to clonidine in hospitalized patients with asymptomatic severe hypertension. Am J Hypertens. 2022;35(5):433-40.
4. Tarkin JM, Kaski JC. Vasodilator therapy: Nitrates and nicorandil. Cardiovasc Drugs Ther. 2016;30(4):367-78.

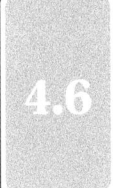

4.6 Newer Therapies for Systemic Hypertension: Renal Denervation Therapy and Baroreceptor Activation Therapy

Ruchit Shah, Srinivasan Narayanan

INTRODUCTION

Systemic hypertension especially if uncontrolled results in major adverse cardiac and cerebral events. Despite multidrug therapy, blood pressures (BPs) are frequently suboptimally controlled and resistant hypertension occurs in 5–20% patients. Moreover, adverse drug effects often interfere with patients' lifestyle and affect drug compliance. Therefore, alternative treatment strategies have been under investigation for systemic hypertension.

ANATOMY AND PHYSIOLOGY OF THE RENAL SYMPATHETIC NERVOUS SYSTEM

The renal sympathetic nervous system affects the BP by two pathways as shown in **Figure 1**. It supplies the kidneys by a rich network of efferent, exclusively noradrenergic, sympathetic fibers located in the adventitia of the renal arteries and returns signals to the central nervous system via afferent sympathetic fibers likewise located in the adventitia.

Efferent stimulation at the kidneys results in tubular sodium retention via adluminal basolateral Na/K adenosine triphosphatase (ATPase) mediated by beta-1 adrenoreceptor, a reduced renal blood flow mediated by alpha-1 adrenoreceptors, and renin release from the juxtaglomerular apparatus mediated by beta 1 adrenoreceptors. These effects influence BP regulation in the short and long-term.

PERCUTANEOUS CATHETER-BASED RENAL DENERVATION

Recently minimally invasive catheter-based renal denervation using radiofrequency (RF) ultrasound or perivascular injection of neurotoxic substances such as alcohol to target renal sympathetic nerves has been introduced into practice for treatment of resistant arterial hypertension. Renal denervation reduces BP and improves BP control rates. However, clinical evidence of renal denervation in effective BP lowering is conflicting (**Box 1**).

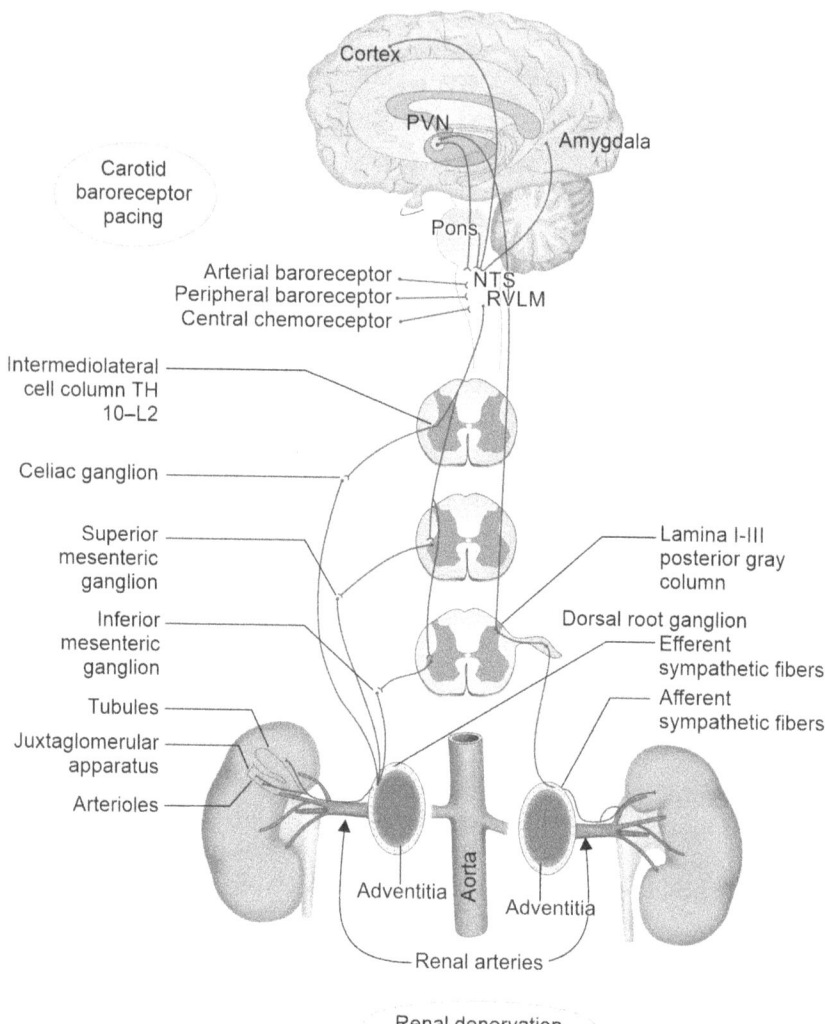

FIG. 1: The renal sympathetic nervous system.
(NTS: nucleus of the solitary tract; PVN: paraventricular nucleus of the hypothalamus; RVLM: rostral ventrolateral medulla)

Box 1: Prerequisites for renal denervation.[1-4]

- Systolic blood pressure ≥160 mm Hg (≥150 mm Hg for type 2 diabetes mellitus)
- ≥3 antihypertensive drugs in adequate dosage and combination (including diuretic)
- Lifestyle modification
- Exclusion of secondary hypertension
- Exclusion of pseudoresistance (ambulatory blood pressure monitoring)
- Preserved renal function (estimated glomerular filtration rate ≥45 mL/min/1.73 m^2)
- Favorable renal anatomy would be a minimal length of 20 mm allowing an adequate landing zone and minimal diameter of 4 mm
- Eligible renal arteries: No stenosis, no percutaneous transluminal angioplasty/stenting

DEVICES AND TECHNIQUES

A renal angiogram is done to assess the anatomy. A special RF catheter **(Fig. 2)** is inserted percutaneously via femoral artery and advanced to the distal segment of the renal artery under fluoroscopy using a guiding catheter. The vessel wall is focally heated up to a maximum of 70°C by means of high frequency energy with a maximum of 8 W for 120 seconds, while the vessel is cooled intraluminally by the high renal blood flow. The focal heating destroys both afferent and efferent sympathetic nerve fibers located in the adventitia. Subsequently, the catheter is pulled back from the distal to proximal vessel segments in steps of minimum 5 mm with rotations in order to capture the entire circumference of the vessel. This results in 4–8 ablations per artery.

Due to the close positioning of the sympathetic nerves and C pain fibers, analog-anesthesia is necessary during the RF ablation procedure.

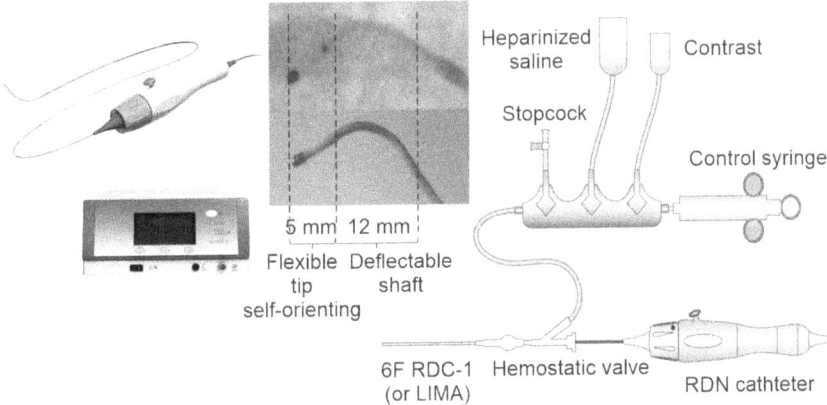

FIG. 2: The symplicity catheter system for renal denervation.
Courtesy: Medtronic Inc.

SAFETY AND LIKELY COMPLICATIONS OF RENAL DENERVATION

Safety
Safety is 98%.

Complications
- Femoral artery pseudoaneurysm
- Renal artery dissection during placement of guiding catheter
- Vasovagal reaction (most common)
- Urinary tract infection and back pain
- Renal artery stenosis
- Sympathetic reinnervation of the kidney in the long-term which may abolish or attenuate the long-term effects of the procedure.

CONTRAINDICATIONS TO RENAL DENERVATION

- Secondary and treatable causes of hypertension
- Anatomical unsuitability of renal arteries (diameter <4 mm; length <20 mm; fibromuscular dysplasia; significant renal artery stenosis)
- Estimated glomerular filtration rate (eGFR) <45 mL/min/1.73 m².

LANDMARK TRIALS OF RENAL DENERVATION THERAPY (TABLE 1)

TABLE 1: Landmark trials of renal denervation therapy.[5,6]

Trial	Comment
SIMPLICITY HTN-1 (n = 45) (2009)	Reduction in SBP/DBP by 14/10 mm Hg at 4 weeks and 27/10 mm Hg at 12 months
SIMPLICITY HTN-2 (n = 24)	BP lowering by 33/19 mm Hg observed
SIMPLICITY HTN-3 (2017)	Failed to show BP reduction at 6 months compared to standard therapy
DENERHTN	Renal denervation + pharmacotherapy better than pharmacotherapy alone
PRAGUE 15	Similar efficacy as DENERHTN, but more side effects with pharmacotherapy
(BP: blood pressure; DBP: diastolic blood pressure; SBP: systolic blood pressure)	

CAROTID BARORECEPTOR ACTIVATION THERAPY FOR RESISTANT HYPERTENSION

Arterial baroreceptors located in the walls of the carotid sinuses and aortic arch are pressure-sensitive nerve endings that sense increase and decrease in BP. Arterial baroreceptors fire when BP raises sending afferent nerve impulses into the central nervous system that reflexively increase parasympathetic outflow inducing bradycardia and peripheral vasodilatation to protect against hypertension there is stiffening of the great vessels in resistant hypertension accompanied by sympathetic overactivity and attenuation of the arterial baroreflex function.

Electrical field stimulation of the carotid baroreceptors using implantable devices has been shown to reduce sympathetic activity and reduce BP in patients with resistant hypertension.

RHEOS PIVOTAL phase III trial on continuous carotid baroreflex activation therapy for resistant hypertension showed equivocal efficacy with surgically induced facial nerve palsy. Miniaturized second-generation systems with unilateral stimulation are undergoing phase III clinical trials in resistant hypertension at present.

CREATING ARTERIOVENOUS FISTULA

An arteriovenous fistula is created between the external iliac artery and vein with the help of a stent-like nitinol device. This has been beneficial in cases of resistant hypertension. Further studies are needed to validate the technique.

FUTURE PERSPECTIVE

Alternative newer modalities using ultrasound and chemical denervation are under study. Surgical resection of the carotid body is also being tried. Device therapy and renal denervation are class III indications with level of evidence B in latest European Society of Cardiology (ESC) 2018 guidelines for hypertension.

SUMMARY

Renal denervation is a promising newer modality of treatment for refractory hypertension despite optimal medications, lifestyle measures with favorable renal anatomy.

Early results of carotid baroreceptor activation with miniature second-generation devices look promising for treatment of refractory hypertension.

MULTIPLE CHOICE QUESTIONS

1. Newer interventional therapies for resistant hypertension are:
   A. External iliac arteriovenous fistula
   B. Renal denervation
   C. Baroreceptor activation therapy
   D. All of the above

2. Interventional therapy for resistant hypertension is approved by ESC 2018 guidelines as:
   A. Class IA level of indication
   B. Class IIa level of indication
   C. Class IIb level of indication
   D. Class III B level of indication

3. Renal denervation is contraindicated in all, except:
   A. Secondary hypertension
   B. Renal artery stenosis
   C. Systolic BP>160 mm Hg on >3 antihypertensives on optimal doses
   D. Resistant hypertension with renal failure

4. Renal denervation involves ablation of:
   A. Afferent fibers
   B. Efferent fibers
   C. Both afferent and efferent fibers
   D. None of the above

5. Minimally invasive catheter based renal denervation uses the following
   A. Radiofrequency
   B. Ultrasound
   C. Perivascular injection
   D. All of the above

Answers

1—D 2—D 3—C 4—C 5—D

REFERENCES

1. Schmieder RE, Mahfoud F, Mancia G, Azizi M, Böhm M, Dimitriadis K, et al. European Society of Hypertension position paper on renal denervation 2021. J Hypertens. 2021 Sep 1;39(9):1733-41.
2. Pisano A, Iannone LF, Leo A, Russo E, Coppolino G, Bolignano D. Renal denervation for resistant hypertension. Cochrane Database Syst Rev. 2021;11(11):CD011499.
3. Gupta A, Prince M, Bob-Manuel T, Jenkins JS. Renal denervation: Alternative treatment options for hypertension? Prog Cardiovasc Dis. 2020;63(1):51-7.
4. Townsend RR, Sobotka PA. Catheter-based renal denervation for hypertension. Curr Hypertens Rep. 2018;20(11):93.
5. Kandzari DE, Mahfoud F, Weber MA, Townsend R, Parati G, Fisher NDL, et al. Clinical trial design principles and outcomes definitions for device-based therapies for hypertension: A consensus document from the Hypertension Academic Research Consortium. Circulation. 2022;145(11):847-63.
6. Rosa J, Widimský P, Waldauf P, Zelinka T, Petrák O, Táborský M, et al. Renal denervation in comparison with intensified pharmacotherapy in true resistant hypertension: 2-year outcomes of randomized PRAGUE-15 study. J Hypertens. 2017;35(5):1093-9.

SUGGESTED READINGS

1. Renal denervation: A phoenix from the ashes? British Cardiovascular Society (BCS) editorial Chris Saunderson.
2. Ewen S, Ukena C, Bohm M, Mahfoud F. Percutaneous renal denervation: new treatment for resistant hypertension and more. Heart. 2013;99:1129-34.
3. Victor RG. Carotid baroreflex activation therapies for resistant hypertension. Nat Rev Cardiol. 2015;12(8):451-63

CHAPTER 5

Special Subsets

Amit A Saraf, Nihar Mehta

5.1: Hypertension in Obesity and Metabolic Syndrome
Amit A Saraf, Nimish Shah

5.2: Hypertension in Special Subsets: Cerebrovascular Disease
Vibhor Pardasani

5.3: Hypertensive Emergency
Anand Bhabhor

5.4: Hypertension and Diabetes
Mitul A Shah

5.5: Hypertension and Heart Failure
Mitul A Shah

5.6: Hypertension and Pregnancy
Anand Bhabhor

5.7: Hypertension in Chronic Kidney Disease
Sudhiranjan Dash Choudhury

5.8: Perioperative Hypertension
Shivani Kamat

5.9: Hypertension in Special Subsets: Ischemic Heart Disease
Ruchit Shah, Nandhakumar Vasu

5.10: Management of Hypertension in Pulmonary Diseases
Nimish Shah

5.11: Resistant Hypertension
Amjad Khan

5.1 Hypertension in Obesity and Metabolic Syndrome

Amit A Saraf, Nimish Shah

INTRODUCTION

Hypertension remains one of the most frequently undiagnosed medical condition until relatively late in its course. Due to the late diagnosis, it often leads to a variety of other life-threatening conditions including chronic kidney disease and heart failure.[1,2]

High blood pressure is a very prominent feature of the metabolic syndrome, present in up to 85% of patients with the condition. In the context of global cardiovascular risk, metabolic syndrome is indeed a high-risk condition which involves obesity, dyslipidemia, hypertension, and diabetes. In spite of various controversies surrounding its definition and etiology, metabolic syndrome represents a useful and simple clinical entity which allows for earlier detection of those at high risk of developing cardiovascular disease and type 2 diabetes mellitus (T2DM) and thus preventing development of full-blown disease by earlier implementation of lifestyle interventions.

The concept of the metabolic syndrome became popular[3] long before the association of elevated blood pressure and metabolic abnormalities with poor cerebrovascular outcome had been recognized. However, the establishment of hypertension as a component of the metabolic syndrome, previously named syndrome X, has facilitated better insight into the condition and allowed for earlier detection and treatment.

The metabolic syndrome refers to the clustering of cardiovascular risk factors that include diabetes, obesity, dyslipidemia, and hypertension. According to the World Health Organization (WHO) definition from 1999, metabolic syndrome is present in a person with diabetes, impaired fasting glucose, impaired glucose tolerance, or insulin resistance harboring at least two of the following criteria: Waist-hip ratio >0.90 cm in men or >0.85 cm in women, serum triglycerides ≥150 mg/dL, or high-density lipoprotein cholesterol (HDL-C) 20 µg/min and blood pressure ≥140/90 mm Hg.[4]

PATHOPHYSIOLOGY

Pathogenesis of hypertension in metabolic syndrome could be caused by a number of genetic and acquired conditions.[5] A few rare cases involving antibodies against insulin receptor or mutations in the insulin receptor gene are the exception as insulin resistance of the metabolic syndrome commonly results from impairments in cellular events distal to the interaction between insulin and its surface receptor.[4,5]

Metabolic abnormalities result from the interaction between the effects of insulin resistance located primarily in muscle and adipose tissue and the adverse impact of the compensatory hyperinsulinemia on tissues that normally remain in an insulin sensitive state.[5]

Insulin resistance and the resulting hyperinsulinemia induce elevation in blood pressure by activation of the sympathetic nervous system and renin–angiotensin aldosterone system (RAAS) with consequential sodium retention and volume expansion, endothelial dysfunction, and alteration in renal function.[5,6] Hyperinsulinemia causes stimulation and the activation of RAAS in cardiovascular system, generating the production of angiotensin II and its proatherogenic effects.

At the same time, in insulin-resistant subjects, hyperinsulinemia stimulates the mitogen-activated protein kinase (MAPK) pathway, which is responsible for vascular and cardiac injury.[6,7] Angiotensin II acts through angiotensin I receptors, it inhibits the vasodilatory effects of insulin on blood vessels and glucose uptake into the skeletal muscle cells by blocking insulin action on phosphatidylinositol 3 kinase and protein kinase beta through free oxygen production.[5,7] This resulting effect is decrease in nitric oxide (NO) production in endothelial cells and vasoconstriction in smooth muscle cells and inhibits glucose transport (GLUT 4) in skeletal muscles.

The other mechanism by which insulin resistance contributes to hypertension is overactivity of angiotensin I receptor, which further causes vasoconstriction and volume expansion.[4,5]

In development of arterial hypertension, increased visceral fat accumulation remains a strong predictor. Sympathetic nervous system overactivation is one of the proposed mechanism by which hypertension and obesity are linked.[2,7-9] Chronic sympathetic stimulation facilitates energy balance and weight stabilization in chronic overeating, but this occurs at the cost of adverse consequences such as elevated blood pressure. For hypertension that accompanies visceral obesity, it has also been suggested that chronic elevation in portal venous fatty acid levels may be responsible. Visceral fat represents a metabolically active organ which is strongly related to insulin sensitivity in comparison to subcutaneous tissue.[2] Visceral adipose tissue is also a production depot for cytokines including tumor necrosis factor alpha (TNF-α), which stimulates interleukin-6 (IL-6) production and further generates the production of C-reactive protein (CRP), fibrinogen, and plasminogen activator inhibitor-1 (PAI-1) resulting in a prothrombotic state. In obese subjects and in diabetic patients, the circulating level of cytokines generally remains elevated.[8] On the contrary, visceral adiposity is a state in which there is a relative deficiency of adiponectin—the adipocyte, which increases insulin sensitivity, glucose uptake in muscle cells, and free fatty acid oxidation. This cytokine exerts antidiabetic, anti-inflammatory, and antiatherogenic effects. Hence, adiponectin was recommended as a marker of arterial hypertension.[2,8]

In conclusion, insulin resistance and central obesity are recognized as the main factors involved in the pathophysiology of the metabolic syndrome, contribute to elevated blood pressure, which further promotes vascular damage in cardiac, renal, and brain tissue. Insulin resistance and the resulting hyperinsulinemia induce blood pressure elevation by the activation of sympathetic nervous system and RAAS with consequential sodium retention and volume expansion, endothelial dysfunction, and alteration in renal function. Visceral fat, in comparison to subcutaneous tissue, represents a metabolically active organ, strongly related to insulin sensitivity. Moderating the secretion of various adipocytokines such as leptin, adiponectin, PAI-1, TNF-α, IL-6, and resistin, it is associated with the processes of inflammation, endothelial dysfunction, hypertension, and atherogenesis. One of the proposed mechanisms by which hypertension is linked with central obesity includes sympathetic nervous system overactivation.[9]

THERAPEUTIC APPROACH TO PATIENTS WITH HYPERTENSION AND METABOLIC SYNDROME

Therapeutic approach in patients with hypertension and metabolic syndrome includes lifestyle intervention as unhealthy lifestyle can aggravate the underlying pathology. This treatment includes sodium restriction, alcohol and calorie restriction, smoking cessation, weight reduction, and increased physical activity. However, it is often not sufficient to obtain the target values.[6,10]

This fact underlines the therapeutic importance of pharmacological interventions capable of reducing blood pressure and other abnormalities related to metabolic syndrome such as dyslipidemia, obesity, and diabetes. Among pharmacological agents, particular emphasis is placed on the RAAS blockade with angiotensin-converting enzyme (ACE) inhibitors and angiotensin II receptor blockers, and central sympatholytic agents that exert additional beneficial effects.[4,5] Evidence has been provided that drugs acting on the renin–angiotensin system should be the drugs of choice considering their sympathetic inhibitory effect and increase in insulin sensitivity.[10]

Central sympatholytic agents have favorable metabolic effects particularly imidazoline drugs are indicated. Drugs of the imidazoline class inhibit sympathetic nervous system outflow from the brain, counteracting one of the pathophysiological abnormalities in hypertensive patients with metabolic syndrome, which is activation of the sympathetic nervous system. Inhibition of the sympathetic outflow to skeletal muscle blood vessels further exerts the beneficial effect of increasing insulin sensitivity.[3]

If T2DM is present, in two-thirds of the target, blood pressure values could be achieved only with the use of two or more antihypertensive drugs.[8,10]

In summation, hypertension is more than just elevated blood pressure, it is intimately associated with the metabolic syndrome. In patients with metabolic syndrome, a multi-target approach involving lifestyle changes and drug therapy based on the assessment of the overall cardiovascular risk should be applied.

SUMMARY

- The metabolic syndrome refers to the clustering of cardiovascular risk factors that include diabetes, obesity, dyslipidemia, and hypertension.
- The association of elevated blood pressure and metabolic abnormalities with poor cerebrovascular outcome had been recognized long before the concept of the metabolic syndrome became popular.
- Insulin resistance and the resulting hyperinsulinemia induce blood pressure elevation by activation of the sympathetic nervous system and RAAS.
- Increased visceral fat accumulation is a strong predictor of arterial hypertension. One of the proposed mechanisms by which hypertension is linked with central obesity includes sympathetic nervous system overactivation.
- Evidence has been provided that drugs acting on the renin–angiotensin system and central sympatholytic agents, particularly imidazoline drugs, should be the drugs of choice considering their sympathetic inhibitory effect and increase in insulin sensitivity.

MULTIPLE CHOICE QUESTIONS

1. Metabolic syndrome involves the following disorders, except:
   A. Dyslipidemia
   B. Diabetes insipidus
   C. Hypertension
   D. Obesity

2. According to WHO definition, metabolic syndrome involves the following blood sugar anomalies:
   A. Impaired glucose tolerance
   B. Insulin resistance
   C. Impaired fasting glucose
   D. All of the above

3. According to WHO definition, diagnostic criteria for metabolic syndrome includes:
   A. Waist–hip ratio >0.9 in men and >0.85 in women
   B. Serum triglycerides ≥150 mg/dL or HDL-C 20 µg/min
   C. Blood pressure ≥140 mm Hg
   D. All of the above

4. Hyperinsulinemia-induced blood pressure elevation involves the following mechanisms, except:
   A. Activation of the sympathetic nervous system
   B. Decreased activity of the angiotensin I receptor
   C. Endothelial dysfunction and alteration in renal function
   D. Sodium retention and volume expansion

5. Among pharmacological agents for hypertension with metabolic syndrome, drugs acting on RAAS are preferred because of:
   A. Sympathetic inhibitory effect
   B. Increase in insulin sensitivity
   C. Both of them
   D. None of the above

Answers

1—B   2—D   3—D   4—B   5—C

REFERENCES

1. Mancia G, De Backer G, Dominiczak A, Cifkova R, Fagard R, Germano G, et al. 2007 Guidelines for the Management of Arterial Hypertension: The Task Force for the Management of Arterial Hypertension of the European Society of Hypertension (ESH) and of the European Society of Cardiology (ESC). J Hypertens. 2007;25:1105-87.
2. Kearney PM, Whelton M, Reynolds K, Mountner P, Whelton PK, He J. Global burden of hypertension: analysis of worldwide data. Lancet. 2005;365:217-23.
3. Kannel WB. Blood pressure as a cardiovascular risk factor: prevention and treatment. JAMA. 1996;275:1571-6.
4. World Health Organization. Definition, diagnosis and classification of diabetes mellitus and its complications. Geneva: WHO; 1999.
5. Expert Panel on Detection, Evaluation, and Treatment of High Blood Cholesterol in Adults. Executive summary of the third report of the National Cholesterol Education Program (NCEP) Expert Panel on Detection and Treatment of High Blood Cholesterol in Adults (Adult Treatment Panel III). JAMA. 2001;285:2468-97.
6. European Society of Hypertension-European Society of Cardiology Guidelines Committee. 2003 European Society of Hypertension – European Society of Cardiology guidelines for the management of arterial hypertension. J Hypertens. 2003;21:1011-53.
7. Chobanian AV, Bakris GL, Black HR, Cushman WC, Green LA, Izzo JL Jr, et al. Seventh report of the Joint National Committee on prevention, detection, evaluation and treatment of high blood pressure. J Hypertens. 2003;42:1206-52.
8. Kannel WB. Framingham study insights into hypertensive risk of cardiovascular disease. Hypertens Res. 1995;18:181-96.
9. The sixth report of the Joint National Committee on prevention, detection, evaluation and treatment of high blood pressure. The sixth report (JNC VI). Arch Intern Med. 1997;157:2413-46.
10. Kjeldsen Sverre E, Naditch-Brule L, Perlini, S, Zidek W, Farsang Csaba E. Increased prevalence of metabolic syndrome in uncontrolled hypertension across Europe: the Global Cardiometabolic Risk Profile in Patients with Hypertension Disease survey. J Hypertens. 2008;26:2064-70.

5.2 Hypertension in Special Subsets: Cerebrovascular Disease

Vibhor Pardasani

INTRODUCTION

Hypertension is a well-established risk factor for cerebrovascular disease. In addition, blood pressure (BP) management determines the outcome of patients with stroke. However, the management varies depending on whether the stroke is ischemic or hemorrhagic as well as whether it is acute or chronic.

ISCHEMIC STROKE

Blood pressure is usually elevated in patients with acute ischemic stroke (AIS). This may be due to chronic hypertension, an acute sympathetic response, or other stroke-mediated mechanisms to protect cerebral perfusion. The acute hypertensive effect is transient, as BP can normalize in a lot of patients within 10 days. In patients with AIS, the cerebral perfusion distal to the obstructed vessel is low. Since cerebral autoregulation gets impaired in acute stroke, blood flow in the dilated distal vessels gets dependent upon the systemic BP. Lowering the BP too rapidly can impair the perfusion and worsen the neurologic deficit.

- If a patient presents with AIS within 4.5 hours of symptom onset, it is mandatory to reduce the systolic blood pressure (SBP) below 185 mm Hg and diastolic blood pressure (DBP) below 110 mm Hg before thrombolytic therapy can be initiated. This reduces the risk of thrombolysis-related intracranial hemorrhage (ICH). BP should be stabilized and maintained at or below 180/105 mm Hg for at least 24 hours after thrombolytic treatment. The same principle also applies to patients with acute large artery thrombosis, who are being considered for mechanical thrombectomy.
- If a patient with AIS is not considered for thrombolytic therapy, BP should be lowered only if it is extreme (SBP >220 mm Hg or DBP >120 mm Hg), or in case of acute coronary syndrome, heart failure, aortic dissection, hypertensive encephalopathy, or preeclampsia/eclampsia. In such patients, BP should be lowered gradually and cautiously by approximately 15% during the first 24 hours after stroke onset.
- For AIS patients with stable neurologic deficit, who remain hypertensive (>140/90 mm Hg) more than 3 days after the event, antihypertensive should be initiated/reintroduced. The BP should be lowered gradually

over 7–14 days in AIS patients with large artery stenoses, proven on carotid Doppler study or on angiogram.
- The choice of antihypertensive drug in this situation and for secondary prevention is guided by the patient profile and the comorbidities. There is no definite evidence suggesting superiority of one antihypertensive class over another.

When immediate antihypertensive therapy is needed, intravenous (IV) agents are recommended owing to the rapid onset of action, short half-lives, and thereby ease of titration. Labetalol is the agent of choice. It is given in a dose of 10–20 mg IV over 2 minutes; can be repeated in double dose (maximum 80 mg/dose) at 10-minute intervals to achieve the target BP; total maximum dose: 300 mg. Alternatively after the initial bolus, a continuous infusion can be started at 0.5–2 mg/min. IV nitroprusside and nitroglycerin are generally avoided since they can potentially elevate the intracranial pressure.

Sublingual nifedipine which is commonly used in general practice for accelerated hypertension can cause a prolonged or precipitous decline in blood pressure which can worsen the neurologic deficit. It should therefore be avoided.

If a patient with AIS is neurologically worsening or is unstable, antihypertensive therapy should be delayed till the stroke-related deficits have stabilized.

ACUTE HEMORRHAGIC STROKE

Blood pressure is generally more elevated in patients with hemorrhagic stroke as compared to ischemic stroke. For patients with acute ICH who present with SBP between 150 and 220 mm Hg, reducing it rapidly (over 6 hours) to 140 mm Hg lowers the risk of hematoma expansion and thereby improves outcome. Unlike in AIS, BP lowering in the perihematomal region does not impair the outcome in ICH. In patients with SBP ≥220 mm Hg, rapid lowering of SBP to <180 mm Hg with IV labetalol is beneficial.

TRANSIENT ISCHEMIC ATTACK

If a patient who has fully recovered from his neurologic deficit has no evidence of acute infarction, antihypertensive therapy should be initiated/reintroduced immediately.

SUBARACHNOID HEMORRHAGE

In patients with spontaneous aneurysmal subarachnoid hemorrhage (SAH), reducing the BP may decrease the risk of hematoma expansion. However, it may also place the patient at an increased risk of cerebral infarction. The optimal therapy in such a situation is not clear. Nor do we have a well-defined BP target. Antihypertensives are therefore administered only if there is a severe elevation in BP in an alert patient with acute SAH. Antihypertensives are generally withheld in patients with severely impaired consciousness.

Lowering the SBP to <160 mm Hg is accepted as a reasonable approach. When urgent BP control is essential, IV labetalol is again preferred. However, since nimodipine is routinely used as a vasodilator to prevent vasospasm after an SAH, IV antihypertensives are generally not needed.

SUMMARY

- Accurate BP management determines the outcome of patients with stroke.
- BP is usually elevated in patients with AIS due to chronic hypertension, an acute sympathetic response, or other stroke-mediated mechanisms to protect cerebral perfusion.
- If a patient presents with AIS within 4.5 hours of symptom onset, it is mandatory to reduce the SBP below 185 mm Hg and DBP below 110 mm Hg before thrombolytic therapy can be initiated.
- If a patient with AIS is not considered for thrombolytic therapy, BP should be lowered only if it is extreme (SBP >220 mm Hg or DBP >120 mm Hg), or in case of hypertensive emergencies.
- For patients with acute ICH who present with SBP between 150 and 220 mm Hg, reducing it rapidly (over 6 hours) to 140 mm Hg lowers the risk of hematoma expansion.
- Antihypertensives are administered only if there is a severe elevation in BP in an alert patient with acute SAH and are generally withheld in patients with severely impaired consciousness.

MULTIPLE CHOICE QUESTIONS

1. In AIS patients, the preferred antihypertensive is:
   A. Nifedipine
   B. Amlodipine
   C. Labetalol
   D. None of the above

2. In AIS patients not receiving thrombolytic therapy, BP should be lowered only in case of:
   A. Acute coronary syndrome
   B. Preeclampsia
   C. Aortic dissection
   D. All of the above

3. In immediate antihypertensive therapy, IV agents are recommended because:
   A. Rapid onset of action
   B. Short half-life
   C. Ease of titration
   D. All of the above

CHAPTER 5 Special Subsets

4. Which of these is a false statement in relation to AIS?
   A. IV nitroprusside is avoided as it may elevate the intracranial pressure
   B. Sublingual nifedipine can cause prolonged decline in BP
   C. In neurologically unstable patients, immediate antihypertensive therapy should be administered
   D. In secondary HTN, the choice of antihypertensive drug depends on patient profile and comorbidities

5. Which of these is a false statement in relation to SAH?
   A. IV labetalol is the preferred antihypertensive drug
   B. Nimodipine is routinely used to prevent vasospasm after an SAH
   C. Both of them
   D. None of the above

Answers

1—C   2—D   3—D   4—C   5—D

SUGGESTED READINGS

1. Powers WJ, Rabinstein AA, Ackerson T, Adeoye OM, Bambakidis NC, Becker K, et al. 2018 guidelines for the early management of patients with acute ischemic stroke: A guideline for healthcare professionals from the American Heart Association/American Stroke Association. Stroke. 2018;49(3):e46-110.
2. Morgenstern LB, Hemphill JC, Anderson C, Becker K, Broderick JP, Connolly ES Jr, et al. Guidelines for the management of spontaneous intracerebral hemorrhage: a guideline for healthcare professionals from the American Heart Association/American Stroke Association. Stroke. 2010;41(9):2108-29.
3. Connolly ES Jr, Rabinstein AA, Carhuapoma JR, Derdeyn CP, Dion J, Higashida RT, et al. Guidelines for the management of aneurysmal subarachnoid hemorrhage: a guideline for healthcare professionals from the American Heart Association/American Stroke Association. Stroke. 2012;43(6):1711-37.

5.3 Hypertensive Emergency

Anand Bhabhor

INTRODUCTION

Severe hypertension is defined when blood pressure exceeds 180/110 mm Hg in the absence of symptoms beyond mild or moderate headache and without evidence of acute target organ damage.

Hypertensive urgency is defined when blood pressure exceeds 180/110 mm Hg in the presence of significant symptoms, such as severe headache or dyspnea, but has nil or only minimal acute target organ damage.

Hypertensive emergency is defined when very high blood pressure (>220/140 mm Hg) is accompanied by evidence of life-threatening organ dysfunction such as cardiac, renal, retinal, or neurological **(Table 1)**.

TABLE 1: Target organ damage.[1,2]

Cardiovascular	• Myocardial infarction • Unstable angina • Aortic dissection • Left ventricular failure
Central nervous system	• Cerebral edema • Altered mental status-encephalopathy • Intracerebral or subarachnoid bleeding
Renal	• Proteinuria • Acute renal failure
Ophthalmologic	• Retinal hemorrhage or exudates • Papilledema

TREATMENT GOAL

Hypertensive Urgency
- *Immediate goal*: Lower blood pressure within 24–72 hours
- *Medication*: Oral medication with rapid onset; occasionally intravenous drugs

Hypertensive Emergency

- *Immediate goal*: Lower BP by 15–20% within 2 hours, 25% within 12 hours, and 30% within 48 hours
- *Medication*: Intravenous

INVESTIGATIONS

- Electrocardiogram (ECG)
- Complete blood count (CBC)
- Renal function test (RFT)
- Liver function test (LFT)
- Thyroid function test (TFT)
- Lipid profile
- Urine examination
- Two-dimensional (2D) ECHO
- X-ray of the chest
- Computed tomography (CT) of the head in neurologic findings are abnormal
- Renal artery Doppler
- Urinary vanillylmandelic acid (VMA)/metanephrines/5-HIAA (hydroxyindoleacetic acid) for pheochromocytoma if clinical suspicion

DRUGS FOR HYPERTENSIVE URGENCY (TABLE 2)

TABLE 2: Drugs for hypertensive urgency.[1-6]

Agent	Dose	Onset of action	Remarks
Captopril	12.5–25 mg PO	15–60 minutes	Can precipitate acute renal failure in patients with bilateral renal artery stenosis
Nifedipine	10–20 mg PO	20 minutes	Avoid short-acting or sublingual nifedipine due to risk of sudden hypotension, stroke, and cardiac event
Labetalol	200–400 mg PO	20–120 minutes	Heart failure, bronchospasm, and bradycardia
Clonidine	0.1–0.2 mg PO	30–60 minutes	Rebound hypertension due to abrupt withdrawal
Prazosin	1–2 mg PO	2–4 hours	First-dose hypotension, syncope, and tachycardia
Amlodipine	5–10 mg PO	30–50 minutes	Headache, tachycardia, and flushing

DRUGS FOR HYPERTENSIVE EMERGENCY (TABLE 3)

TABLE 3: Drugs for hypertensive emergency.

Agents	Dose	Onset of action	Remarks
Sodium nitroprusside	0.25–10 µg/kg/min IV infusion	Onset: Seconds Duration of action: 2–3 minutes	• Infusion bag and delivery set must be light resistant or covered • Thiocyanate/cyanide intoxication, metabolic acidosis in patients with renal impairment • Thiocyanate level >10 mg/dL should be avoided
Nitroglycerin	5–100 µg/min IV infusion	Onset: 2–5 minutes Duration of action: 5–15 minutes	• Headache, tachycardia, flushing, vomiting • Develops tolerance with use • Useful in cardiac failure or ischemia
Labetalol	10–80 mg IV bolus every 10 minutes to a maximum dose of 300 mg Infusion: 0.5–2 mg/min	Onset: 5–10 minutes Duration of action: 3–6 hours	• Bradycardia, bronchospasm • Avoid in congestive heart failure, bronchial asthma • Commonly use in pregnancy induced hypertension
Enalapril	1.25 mg every 6 hours	Onset: 15–30 minutes Duration of action: 6–12 hours	• Contraindicated in pregnancy and renal artery stenosis • Useful in patient with congestive heart failure
Esmolol	500 µg/kg IV bolus and can be repeated after 5 minutes Infusion: 50–200 µg/kg/min	Onset: 1–5 minutes Duration of action: 15–30 minutes	• Avoid in CHF, heart block, and asthma
Hydralazine	10–20 mg IV boluses may be repeated every 30 minutes till target BP is achieved or unacceptable tachycardia develops	Onset: 10–30 minutes Duration of action: 2–4 hours	• Reflex tachycardia, flushing • Avoid in patients with raised ICP, IHD, and aortic dissection (without beta-blocker)

Continued

Continued

Agents	Dose	Onset of action	Remarks
Phentolamine	5–15 mg IV bolus, repeat every 5–15 minutes *Infusion*: 0.2–5 mg/min		• Reflex tachycardia • Postural hypotension • Useful in Pheochromocytoma
Nicardipine	5 mg/h IV infusion; titrate up by 2.5 mg/h every 20 minutes to maximum 15 mg/h	*Onset*: 15–30 minutes *Duration of action*: 1–4 hours	• Reflex tachycardia • Avoid in heart failure • Useful in subarachnoid hemorrhage

(BP: blood pressure; CHF: congestive heart failure; ICP: intracranial pressure; IHD: ischemic heart disease; IV: intravenous)

SPECIFIC SITUATION

Pregnancy-induced Hypertension

Posterior reversible encephalopathy syndrome (PRES) is a specific hypertensive emergency during pregnancy.

Drugs of choice: Labetalol, methyldopa, hydralazine, and magnesium sulfate

Neurologic Hypertensive Emergency

Labetalol and calcium channel blocker are preferred in such conditions.
 Nitroglycerin and nitroprusside should be avoided because they may worsen cerebral perfusion.

Acute Aortic Dissection

Blood pressure should be reduced to <120 mm Hg within 20 minutes. β-blocker such as labetalol and esmolol as well as sodium nitroprusside along with β-blocker can be used.

Acute Coronary Syndrome

Nitroglycerin, β-blockers, and angiotensin-converting enzyme (ACE) inhibitors are preferred.

Acute Pulmonary Edema

Nitroglycerin, diuretics, and ACE inhibitors are preferred.

Renal Emergency

- Sodium nitroprusside and labetalol are useful agents.
- Short-term dialysis may sometimes be needed.

Adrenergic Crisis

For example, pheochromocytoma crisis, cocaine, or amphetamine intoxication and patient on monoamine oxidase (MAO) inhibitors ingesting tyramine containing foods.

Pure alpha-blocker such as phentolamine is preferred.

A β-blocker can be added if additional antihypertensive effect is needed.

SUMMARY

- Severe hypertension is defined when blood pressure exceeds 180/110 mm Hg in the absence of significant symptoms and without evidence of acute target organ damage.
- Hypertensive urgency is defined when blood pressure exceeds 180/110 mm Hg in the presence of significant symptoms but has nil or only minimal acute target organ damage.
- Hypertensive emergency is defined when very high blood pressure (>220/140 mm Hg) is accompanied by evidence of life-threatening organ dysfunction
- Investigations should be carried out immediately in order to diagnose and assess the severity of organ damage.
- Nitroglycerin and nitroprusside should be avoided in neurological hypertensive emergency as they may worsen cerebral perfusion.
- Labetalol is the preferred drug of choice in pregnancy-induced hypertension.
- In adrenergic crisis, pure alpha-blocker like phentolamine is preferred.

MULTIPLE CHOICE QUESTIONS

1. HTN-induced ophthalmological damage includes the following, except:
    A. Retinal hemorrhage
    B. Retinal exudate
    C. Papilledema
    D. Retinitis pigmentosa

2. Nitroglycerin has the following side effect:
    A. Headache
    B. Tachycardia
    C. Vomiting
    D. All of the above

3. Antihypertensives contraindicated in renal artery stenosis include:
    A. Enalapril
    B. Captopril
    C. Both of them
    D. None of the above

4. Labetalol is contraindicated in the following, except:
   A. Congestive heart failure
   B. Pregnancy-induced hypertension
   C. Bradycardia
   D. Bronchial asthma
5. The following cause reflex tachycardia:
   A. Hydralazine
   B. Phentolamine
   C. Nicardipine
   D. All of the above

Answers

1—D   2—D   3—C   4—B   5—D

REFERENCES

1. Talle MA, Ngarande E, Doubell AF, Herbst PG. Cardiac complications of hypertensive emergency: Classification, diagnosis and management challenges. J Cardiovasc Dev Dis. 2022;9(8):276.
2. van der Veen PH, Geerlings MI, Visseren FLJ, Nathoe HM, Mali WPTM, van der Graaf Y, et al. Hypertensive target organ damage and longitudinal changes in brain structure and function. The Second Manifestations of Arterial Disease–Magnetic Resonance Study. 2015;66:1152-8.
3. Tocci G, Figliuzzi I, Presta V, Miceli F, Citoni B, Coluccia R, et al. Therapeutic approach to hypertension urgencies and emergencies during acute coronary syndrome. High Blood Press Cardiovasc Prev. 2018;25(3):253-9.
4. Padilla Ramos A, Varon J. Current and newer agents for hypertensive emergencies. Curr Hypertens Rep. 2014;16(7):450.
5. Manning L, Robinson TG, Anderson CS. Control of blood pressure in hypertensive neurological emergencies. Curr Hypertens Rep. 2014;16(6):436.
6. Papadopoulos DP, Sanidas EA, Viniou NA, Gennimata V, Chantziara V, Barbetseas I, et al. Cardiovascular hypertensive emergencies. Curr Hypertens Rep. 2015;17(2):5.

SUGGESTED READINGS

1. Lobanova I, Qureshi AI. Blood pressure goals in acute stroke-how low do you go? Curr Hypertens Rep. 2018;20(4):28.
2. Ahmed N, Wahlgren N, Brainin M, Castillo J, Ford GA, Kaste M, et al. Relationship of blood pressure, antihypertensive therapy, and outcome in ischemic stroke treated with intravenous thrombolysis: retrospective analysis from Safe Implementation of Thrombolysis in Stroke-International Stroke Thrombolysis Register (SITS-ISTR). Stroke. 2009;40(7):2442-9.
3. Balahura AM, Moroi ȘI, Scafa-Udriște A, Weiss E, Japie C, Bartoș D, et al. The management of hypertensive emergencies-is there a "magical" prescription for all? J Clin Med. 2022;11(11):3138.
4. van den Born BH, Lip GYH, Brguljan-Hitij J, Cremer A, Segura J, Morales E, et al. ESC Council on hypertension position document on the management of hypertensive emergencies. Eur Heart J Cardiovasc Pharmacother. 2019;5(1):37-46.

5.4 Hypertension and Diabetes

Mitul A Shah

INTRODUCTION

Diabetes mellitus is defined as a disorder of the metabolic system in which the body does not produce enough insulin or respond normally to insulin, causing abnormal elevation of blood glucose levels and characterized by symptoms such as increased thirst, urination, weight loss, and increased hunger. As per the American Diabetes Association (ADA) 2019 guidelines, an individual is considered to have diabetes mellitus when: Glycosylated hemoglobin (HbA1c) which is the 3-month average blood glucose level also known as HbA1c >6.5% or fasting plasma glucose >126 mg/dL or 2-hour postprandial plasma glucose >200 mg/dL.[1]

Acute complications of diabetes may include:
- Diabetic ketoacidosis
- Hyperosmolar hyperglycemic state
- Sepsis or death
- Chronic complications include:
- Cardiovascular disease
- Stroke
- Chronic kidney disease
- Peripheral vascular disease
- Neuropathy
- Retinopathy
- Cognitive impairment[2]

Microvascular complications caused by diabetes mellitus include diabetic retinopathy, diabetic nephropathy, and diabetic neuropathy.

Macrovascular complications caused by diabetes mellitus include cardiovascular conditions such as ischemic heart disease, peripheral artery disease especially atherosclerotic occlusion of the lower limbs, renovascular conditions, and cerebrovascular accidents (CVAs) (stroke) or transient ischemic attack (TIA). Diabetes mellitus and hypertension are common diseases that generally coexist at a greater frequency than prediction by chance alone.

The risk and acceleration in the course of complications such as cardiovascular diseases, peripheral vascular disease, stroke, retinopathy, and nephropathy markedly increase if hypertension is diagnosed in a diabetic patient.[3]

PATHOPHYSIOLOGY OF HYPERTENSION IN DIABETICS

Pathogenic mechanisms for microvascular complications in diabetes mellitus are as follows:
- The pathologic effects of advanced glycation end products (AGE) accumulation overproduction of endothelial growth factors
- Abnormal stimulation of the protein kinase C (PKC), polyol pathways and the renin-angiotensin system (RAS).

Mechanisms for macrovascular disease in diabetes are as follows:
- The pathologic effects of AGE accumulation, nitric oxide (NO) inhibition causes impaired vasodilatory response, increased production of endothelial growth factors
- Chronic vascular inflammation
- Hemodynamic dysregulation, dysfunction of the smooth muscle cell, impairment in the fibrinolytic ability
- Increased platelet aggregation[4]

Diabetic nephropathy is an important factor, especially in patients with type 1 diabetes mellitus (T1DM) involved in the development of hypertension. However, the underlying renal disease still cannot explain the occurrence of hypertension in a large number of diabetic patients and remains "essential" in nature. Both diabetes mellitus and hypertension share a few common risk factors which include nonmodifiable risk factors such as genetic predisposition, increasing age, and sex. The modifiable risk factors include diet and sedentary lifestyle, obesity, smoking, high cholesterol, and existing cardiovascular and peripheral vascular conditions. However, in spite of the associated risk factors, the hallmark pathological factor of hypertension in both type 1 and type 2 diabetics seems to be an increase in the peripheral vascular resistance. Research also shows that insulin resistance/hyperinsulinemia and increased exchangeable sodium may play key roles in the pathogenesis of hypertension not only in diabetics but in prediabetic individuals as well.[3]

APPROACH TO TREATMENT OF HYPERTENSION IN DIABETICS

The goal of antihypertensive therapy in a diabetic individual is not only to control blood pressure (BP) and reduce it down to a target range but also to minimize the increased cardiovascular risks associated with diabetes and hypertension.
- The initiation of antihypertensive drug treatment in an individual with diabetes is recommended when office BP exceeds 140 mm Hg systolic blood pressure (SBP)/90 mm Hg diastolic blood pressure (DBP).[5]
- The BP goal is to target SBP to 130 mm Hg and <130 mm Hg if tolerated, but not <120 mm Hg. In older people (aged >65 years), the SBP goal is to a range of 130–139 mm Hg.
- It is recommended that DBP is targeted to <80 mm Hg, but not <70 mm Hg.
- An on-treatment SBP of <130 mm Hg may be considered in patients at particularly high risk of a cerebrovascular event, such as those with a history of CVA.

- Lifestyle changes [weight loss if overweight, physical activity, alcohol restriction, sodium restriction, and increased consumption of fruits (e.g., two to three servings), vegetables (e.g., two to three servings), and low-fat dairy products] are highly recommended and should be strictly followed in diabetic and prediabetic patients.
- The use of a renin–angiotensin aldosterone system (RAAS) blocker [angiotensin-converting enzyme (ACE) inhibitors or angiotensin receptor blocker (ARB)] is recommended for diabetic individuals, particularly in those who present with proteinuria including microalbuminuria and albuminuria and cardiac patients with left ventricular (LV) hypertrophy although all other BP-lowering drugs can also be used.
- The recommendation for the initial treatment is combination of a RAAS blocker with a calcium channel blocker or thiazide/thiazide-like diuretic.
- The use of beta-blocker with a diuretic favors the development of diabetes mellitus and should be avoided in prediabetes mellitus, unless no other options are available or the drug is required for other reasons. Hence, RAAS blockers are preferred to beta-blockers or diuretics in patients with impaired fasting glucose (IFG) or impaired glucose tolerance (IGT), in order to reduce the risk of developing diabetes mellitus.
- Nebivolol is the preferred beta-blocker of choice in diabetics as studies show that it does not affect insulin sensitivity in patients with metabolic syndrome.[6]

SUMMARY (TABLE 1)

TABLE 1: Treatment strategies in people with diabetes.

Recommendations	Class[a]	Level[b]
Antihypertensive drug treatment is recommended for people with diabetes when office BP is ≥140/90 mm Hg	I	A
In people with diabetes receiving BP-lowering drugs, it is recommended: • To target SBP to 130 mm Hg and <130 mm Hg if tolerated, but not <120 mm Hg	I	A
• In older people (aged ≥65 years), to target to an SBP range of 130–139 mm Hg	I	A
• To target the DBP to <80 mm Hg, but not <70 mm Hg	I	C
It is recommended to initiate treatment with a combination of a RAS blocker with a CCB or thiazide/thiazide-like diuretic[c]	I	A
Simultaneous administration of two RAS blockers, e.g., an ACE inhibitor and ARB, is not indicated	III	A

[a]Class of recommendation.
[b]Level of evidence.
[c]When eGFR <30 mL/min/1.73 m². Avoid thiazide/thiazide-like diuretics and consider using a loop diuretic when a diuretic is required.
(ACE: angiotensin-converting enzyme; ARB: angiotensin receptor blocker; BP: blood pressure; CCB: calcium channel blacker; DBP: diastolic blood pressure; eGFR: estimated glomerular filtration rate; RAS: renin-angiotensin system; SBP: systolic blood pressure).

MULTIPLE CHOICE QUESTIONS

1. Acute complications of diabetes mellitus include the following, except:
   A. Stroke
   B. Diabetic ketoacidosis
   C. Hyperosmolar hyperglycemic state
   D. Death
2. Microvascular complications of diabetes mellitus include:
   A. Retinopathy
   B. Peripheral vascular disease
   C. Both
   D. None
3. Pathogenic mechanism for macrovascular complications in diabetes mellitus include the following, except:
   A. Smooth muscle cell dysfunction
   B. Overproduction of endothelial growth factors
   C. Chronic inflammation
   D. Abnormal stimulation of protein kinase C
4. The following antihypertensive drugs can be used in diabetes mellitus, except:
   A. ACE inhibitors
   B. ARB
   C. CCB
   D. Beta-blocker
5. The etiology of hypertension in diabetic patients can either be:
   A. Increased exchangeable sodium
   B. Increased peripheral vascular resistance
   C. Insulin resistance
   D. All of the above

Answers

1—A   2—A   3—D   4—D   5—D

REFERENCES

1. American Diabetes Association. 2. Classification and diagnosis of diabetes: Standards of medical care in diabetes-2019. Diabetes Care. 2019;42:S13-28.
2. Saedi E, Gheini MR, Faiz F, Arami MA. Diabetes mellitus and cognitive impairments. World J Diabetes. 2016;7(17):412-22.
3. Epstein M, Sowers J. Diabetes mellitus and hypertension. Hypertension. 1992;19(5):403-18.
4. Cade W. Diabetes-related microvascular and macrovascular diseases in the physical therapy setting. Phys Ther. 2008;88(11):1322-35.
5. Williams B, Mancia G, Spiering W, Agabiti Rosei E, Azizi M, Burnier M, et al. 2018 ESC/ESH guidelines for the management of arterial hypertension. Eur Heart J. 2018;39(33):3021-104.
6. Cosentino F, Grant P, Aboyans V, Bailey C, Ceriello A, Delgado V, et al. 2019 ESC guidelines on diabetes, pre-diabetes, and cardiovascular diseases developed in collaboration with the EASD. Eur Heart J. 2019;41(2):255-323.

5.5 Hypertension and Heart Failure

Mitul A Shah

INTRODUCTION

Heart failure (HF) is a clinical syndrome with symptoms and/or signs caused by a structural and/or functional cardiac abnormality and corroborated by elevated natriuretic peptide levels and/or objective evidence of pulmonary or systemic congestion.[1] This clinical syndrome may lead to development of cardinal symptoms (e.g., breathlessness, ankle swelling, and fatigue) which may be accompanied by signs (e.g., elevated jugular venous pressure, pulmonary crackles, and peripheral edema).[2] HF results in elevated intracardiac pressures and/or inadequate cardiac output at rest and/or during exercise.

TERMINOLOGY AND NEW YORK HEART ASSOCIATION CLASSIFICATION

Heart failure with left ventricular ejection fraction (LVEF) ≤40% is designated as heart failure with reduced ejection fraction (HFrEF), HF with an LVEF between 41 and 49% is designated as heart failure with mildly reduced ejection fraction (HFmrEF), while HF with LVEF ≥50% is designated as heart failure with preserved ejection fraction (HFpEF).[2]

The New York Heart Association (NYHA) functional classification is the commonly used classification to describe the severity of HF **(Table 1)**.

TABLE 1: New York Heart Association (NYHA) classification for heart failure.

Class I	No limitation of physical activity. Ordinary physical activity does not cause undue breathlessness, fatigue, or palpitations
Class II	Slight limitation of physical activity. Comfortable at rest, but ordinary physical activity results in undue breathlessness, fatigue, or palpitations
Class III	Marked limitation of physical activity. Comfortable at rest, but less than ordinary physical activity results in undue breathlessness, fatigue, or palpitations
Class IV	Unable to carry on any physical activity without discomfort. Symptoms at rest can be present. If any physical activity is undertaken, discomfort is increased

ASSOCIATION OF HYPERTENSION WITH HEART FAILURE

Hypertension is a leading risk factor for development of HF. Almost two-thirds of HF patients are known to have hypertension.[3,4] As a consequence of coronary artery disease (CAD), hypertension can lead to HFrEF. Hypertension also causes left ventricular hypertrophy (LVH), which impairs LV relaxation (diastolic dysfunction) and is a potent predictor of HF, even when LV systolic function is normal and there is no preceding myocardial infarction (HFpEF).[5] Hypertension may lead to fibrosis and structural alteration of large and small arteries (microvascular disease) which also contributes to the pathophysiology of development of HF.

Treatment of hypertension has a major impact on reducing the risk of incident HF and HF hospitalization. While diuretics, beta-blockers, angiotensin-converting enzyme (ACE) inhibitors, or angiotensin receptor blockers (ARBs) are the mainstay of therapy, calcium channel blockers (CCBs) have been observed less effective in comparative trials.[6]

Reduction of blood pressure can also lead to the regression of LVH, which has been shown to be accompanied by a reduction of cardiovascular events and mortality. The ARBs, ACE inhibitors, and CCBs cause more effective LVH regression than beta-blockers or diuretics.[5]

MANAGEMENT OF HYPERTENSION IN ACUTE HEART FAILURE

Although most acute heart failure (AHF) patients present with hypotension or borderline pressures, few subsets do have accelerated blood pressure associated with pulmonary edema.

Intravenous diuretics (furosemide or torasemide) are the cornerstone of therapy along with intravenous vasodilators (nitrates or nitroprusside) in these patients.

Diuretics increase renal excretion of salt and water and are indicated for the treatment of fluid overload and congestion in the majority of AHF patients.

The vasodilators dilate venous and arterial vessels leading to a reduction in venous return to the heart, reduction in congestion, lowered afterload, increased stroke volume, and consequent relief of symptoms. Nitrates act mainly on peripheral veins, whereas nitroprusside is more a balanced arterial and venous dilator.

MANAGEMENT OF HYPERTENSION IN CHRONIC HEART FAILURE

If not already initiated, antihypertensive drug treatment should be started when BP is >140/90 mm Hg in patients with HFrEF. The target BP is not defined in patients with HF and needs individualization of treatment. Since poor outcomes are associated with very low BP in HF, it may be wise to avoid actively lowering BP to <120/70 mm Hg. However, some patients may achieve even lower BP levels than this because of the desire to remain on treatment with guideline-directed HF medications, which, if tolerated, should be continued because of their protective effect.[5]

Treatment of HFrEF is similar in hypertensive and normotensive patients. HF guideline-directed medications are recommended for the treatment of hypertension in patients with HFrEF. ACE inhibitors, ARBs, beta-blockers, and mineralocorticoid receptor antagonists (MRAs) (e.g., spironolactone and eplerenone) are all effective in improving clinical outcomes in patients with HFrEF. Diuretics are useful for symptomatic improvement. If further BP lowering is required, a dihydropyridine CCB may be considered. Sacubitril/valsartan has also been shown to improve outcomes in patients with HFrEF and is indicated for the treatment of HFrEF as an alternative to ACE inhibitors or ARBs. Nondihydropyridine CCBs (diltiazem and verapamil), alpha-blockers, and centrally acting agents, such as moxonidine, should not be used.[5]

Antihypertensive treatment is commonly needed in patients with HFpEF with the same BP thresholds and targets as mentioned above.

SUMMARY

- Diuretics and vasodilators are mainstay of treatment of AHF.
- Guideline-directed medical therapy (GDMT) for CHF generally leads to adequate control of hypertension. If still BP is high (>140/90 mm Hg), dihydropyridine CCB can be added.
- ACE inhibitors, ARBs, beta-blockers, MRAs, and angiotensin receptor neprilysin inhibitor (ARNI) (sacubitril/valsartan) are all effective in management of HF as well as control of BP. Diuretics are useful in symptomatic relief.
- Nondihydropyridine CCBs (diltiazem and verapamil), alpha-blockers, and centrally acting agents such as moxonidine should be avoided in treatment of HFrEF.

MULTIPLE CHOICE QUESTIONS

1. Hypertension can lead to development of the following cardiovascular anomalies:
   A. HFrEF
   B. LVH
   C. Microvascular disease
   D. All of the above

2. In hypertensives with acute heart failure, following therapy is preferred:
   A. IV furosemide with IV nitrate
   B. IV furosemide with sublingual nitrate
   C. IV furosemide with oral torasemide
   D. IV furosemide with oral nitroprusside

CHAPTER 5 Special Subsets

3. The action of vasodilators includes the following:
   A. Reduction in venous return to heart
   B. Lowered afterload
   C. Increase stroke volume
   D. All of the above

4. The following can be used in chronic heart failure, except:
   A. Sacubitril/Valsartan
   B. Dihydropyridine
   C. Diltiazem
   D. Spironolactone

5. Acute heart failure can show the following presentation:
   A. Hypotension
   B. Hypertension
   C. Pulmonary edema
   D. All of the above

Answers

1—D   2—A   3—D   4—C   5—D

REFERENCES

1. Bozkurt B, Coats A, Tsutsui H, Abdelhamid M, Adamopoulos S, Albert N, et al. Universal definition and classification of heart failure. J Card Fail. 2021;27(4):387-413.
2. McDonagh T, Metra M, Adamo M, Gardner R, Baumbach A, Böhm M, et al. 2021 ESC Guidelines for the diagnosis and treatment of acute and chronic heart failure. Eur Heart J. 2021;42(36):3599-726.
3. Crespo-Leiro M, Anker S, Maggioni A, Coats A, Filippatos G, Ruschitzka F, et al. European Society of Cardiology Heart Failure Long-Term Registry (ESC-HF-LT): 1-year follow-up outcomes and differences across regions. Eur J Heart Fail. 2016;18(6):613-25.
4. Rapsomaniki E, Timmis A, George J, Pujades-Rodriguez M, Shah A, Denaxas S, et al. Blood pressure and incidence of twelve cardiovascular diseases: lifetime risks, healthy life-years lost, and age-specific associations in 1·25 million people. Lancet. 2014;383(9932):1899-911.
5. Williams B, Mancia G, Spiering W, Agabiti Rosei E, Azizi M, Burnier M, et al. 2018 ESC/ESH Guidelines for the management of arterial hypertension. Eur Heart J. 2018;39(33):3021-104.
6. Thomopoulos C, Parati G, Zanchetti A. Effects of blood pressure-lowering treatment. 6. Prevention of heart failure and new-onset heart failure – meta-analyses of randomized trials. J Hypertens. 2016;34(3):373-84.

5.6 Hypertension and Pregnancy

Anand Bhabhor

CLASSIFICATION

Gestational Hypertension
Hypertension occurring for the first time after 20 weeks of gestation without proteinuria.

Preeclampsia
Hypertension with proteinuria of >0.3 g/24 hours or urine albumin/creatinine ratio >30 mg/mmol after 20 weeks of gestation in a previously nonproteinuric female.

Eclampsia
Preeclampsia with convulsion

Chronic Hypertension Preceding Pregnancy
Blood pressure (BP) >140/90 mm Hg before pregnancy or before 20 weeks of gestation and persists beyond 42 weeks postpartum.

Chronic Hypertension with Superimposed Eclampsia and Preeclampsia
Proteinuria, sudden increase in BP, thrombocytopenia, and abnormal liver enzymes in a previously known hypertensive patient.

COMPLICATIONS OF HYPERTENSION DURING PREGNANCY (TABLE 1)

TABLE 1: Complications of hypertension during pregnancy.[1-3]

Organ system	Clinical signs and symptoms
Cardiovascular	• Hypertension • Pulmonary edema • Reduced CO

Continued

Continued

Organ system	Clinical signs and symptoms
Renal	• Reduced GFR • Proteinuria • Renal cortical necrosis
Central nervous system	• Cerebral hemorrhage, headache/blurred vision Scotoma • Cortical blindness • PRES • Seizures
HELLP	• Elevated liver enzymes • Hepatic dysfunction • Subcapsular bleeding • Hepatic rupture

(CO: cardiac output; GFR: glomerular filtration rate; HELLP: hemolysis, elevated liver enzymes, low platelet count; PRES: posterior reversible encephalopathy syndrome)

WHEN TO START TREATMENT? (TABLE 2)

TABLE 2: Antihypertensive drug in pregnancy.[4-7]

Group	Molecule	Benefit	Side effect
Class	Agent	Effect	Side effect
Calcium channel blocker			
Preferred	Nifedipine[6]	Lowers BP without altering umbilical arterial blood flow	Fetal distress, profound hypotension with magnesium
Alternative	Verapamil[4]	Similar efficacy to other agents	Untested safety profile
Direct vasodilator			
Preferred	Hydralazine[4]	Most efficacious oral agent	Maternal neuropathy, drug induced lupus, and neonatal thrombocytopenia
Alternative	Nitroprusside[4]	Efficacious in severe hypertension	Cyanide and thiocyanate toxicity
Central agent			
Preferred	Methyldopa[6]	Proven safety and efficacy	Neurodepressant side effect
Alternative	Clonidine[5]	Efficacy similar to methyldopa	Unproven safety

Continued

Continued

Group / Class	Molecule / Agent	Benefit / Effect	Side effect
Beta-blocker	Labetalol[7]	Similar to methyldopa	Fetal bradycardia, neonatal hypoglycemia, and decreased placental flow
Diuretics	Thiazide [5]	Useful in chronic HT, kidney failure and congestive heart failure	Volume contraction and electrolyte abnormality
Drugs contraindicated in pregnancy			
Beta-blocker	Atenolol[4]		Intrauterine growth retardation
Diuretics	Spironolactone[5]		Possible fetal antiandrogen effect
RAAS blockage	ACE inhibitor/ ARBs[4]		Associated with congenital heart and kidney diseases

(ACE: angiotensin-converting enzyme; ARB: angiotensin receptor blocker; BP: blood pressure; RAAS: renin–angiotensin–aldosterone system)

- All women with persistent elevation of BP >155/95 mm Hg
- At value >140/90 mm Hg in women with following:
    - Gestational hypertension with or without proteinuria
    - Preexisting hypertension with superimposition of gestational hypertension
    - Hypertension with subclinical organ damage

COMMON AGENTS USED TO TREAT HYPERTENSION

- *Methyldopa*: 250–500 mg orally two to four times daily (maximum 2 g)
- *Labetalol*: 100–400 mg orally two to four times daily (maximum 1,200 mg)
- *Nifedipine*: 10–20 mg orally two to three times daily (maximum 80 mg)

TREATMENT OF ACCELERATED HYPERTENSION IN PREGNANCY (TABLE 3)

TABLE 3: Treatment of accelerated hypertension in pregnancy.

Agent	Dosage
Labetalol	Start with 20 mg IV slowly over 10 minutes; repeat 20–80 mg after 30 minutes if no response
	Or
	Infusion @1–2 mg/kg/min up to maximum of 300 mg

Continued

Agent	Dosage
Nifedipine	5–10 mg capsule bitten and swallowed every 30 minutes Or 10 mg PA tablet every 45 minutes to maximum 80 mg in a day
Hydralazine	Start with 2–5 mg IV and increase dose up to 10 mg every 30 minutes Or Infusion @0.5–10 mg/hr to maximum 20 mg
(IV: intravenous)	

TREATMENT OF ECLAMPSIA

- Magnesium sulfate is crucial in prevention of seizure in patient of preeclampsia by slowing the neuromuscular conduction and raising the seizure threshold.
- Loading dose of magnesium sulfate 4-6 g diluted in 100 mL normal saline and infused over 15-20 minutes, followed by continuous infusion at 2 g/h.
- Continuous monitoring for sign of magnesium toxicity has to be observed, e.g., loss of deep tendon reflex, respiratory depression, and mental status changes.
- Monitor serum magnesium level frequently, target therapeutic range is 4-6 mg/dL.
- In case of toxicity, administer injection calcium gluconate 10% diluted in 10 mL saline slowly over 10 minutes.
- Seizure prophylaxis should continue 12-24 hours postpartum.

SUMMARY

- Hypertension in pregnancy is classified as gestational hypertension, preeclampsia, eclampsia, chronic hypertension preceding pregnancy, and chronic hypertension with superimposed preeclampsia.
- It is associated with cardiac, central nervous system (CNS), hepatic, renal, and hematological complications.
- Treatment is started in all women with persistent elevation of BP >155/95 mm Hg or at value >140/90 mm Hg in women with gestational hypertension with/without proteinuria and hypertension with subclinical organ damage.
- The preferred agents are beta-blockers, calcium channel blockers, thiazide diuretics, and centrally acting antihypertensives. IV is the preferred modality for precise and rapid control of BP.
- Magnesium sulfate stands at the center of management of eclampsia. Monitoring of deep tendon reflex (DTR), respiratory rate, and mental status changes is mandatory to avert magnesium toxicity.

MULTIPLE CHOICE QUESTIONS

1. HELLP (hemolysis, elevated liver enzymes, low platelet count) syndrome involves the following pathological mechanisms:
   A. Hemolysis
   B. Elevated liver enzymes
   C. Low platelet count
   D. All of the above

2. Following are contraindicated in pregnancy except:
   A. Atenolol
   B. Spironolactone
   C. Nifedipine
   D. Captopril

3. Antihypertensive treatment in pregnancy should be started in the following:
   A. Persistent elevation of BP > 155/95 mm Hg
   B. Gestational HTN with BP > 140/90 mm Hg without proteinuria
   C. Both of them
   D. None of the above

4. Labetalol shows the following side effects, except:
   A. Fetal bradycardia
   B. Neonatal hypoglycemia
   C. Decreased placental flow
   D. Intrauterine growth retardation

5. Signs of magnesium toxicity include:
   A. Loss of deep tendon reflex
   B. Respiratory depression
   C. Altered mental status
   D. All of the above

Answers

1—D   2—C   3—C   4—D   5—D

REFERENCES

1. Braunthal S, Brateanu A. Hypertension in pregnancy: Pathophysiology and treatment. SAGE Open Med. 2019;7:2050312119843700.
2. von Dadelszen P, Menzies J, Magee LA. The complications of hypertension in pregnancy. Minerva Med. 2005;96(4):287-302.
3. Seely EW, Ecker J. Chronic hypertension in pregnancy. Circulation. 2014;129(11):1254-61.
4. Tita AT, Szychowski JM, Boggess K, Dugoff L, Sibai B, Lawrence K, et al. Chronic Hypertension and Pregnancy (CHAP) Trial Consortium. Treatment for mild chronic hypertension during pregnancy. N Engl J Med. 2022;386(19):1781-92.

5. Greene MF, Williams WW. Treating hypertension in pregnancy. N Engl J Med. 2022;386(19):1846-7.
6. Easterling T, Mundle S, Bracken H, Parvekar S, Mool S, Magee LA, et al. Oral antihypertensive regimens (nifedipine retard, labetalol, and methyldopa) for management of severe hypertension in pregnancy: an open-label, randomised controlled trial. Lancet. 2019;394(10203):1011-21.
7. Shekhar S, Sharma C, Thakur S, Verma S. Oral nifedipine or intravenous labetalol for hypertensive emergency in pregnancy: a randomized controlled trial. Obstet Gynecol. 2013;122(5):1057-63.

SUGGESTED READINGS

1. Duley L, Gülmezoglu AM, Henderson-Smart DJ, Chou D. Magnesium sulphate and other anticonvulsants for women with pre-eclampsia. Cochrane Database Syst Rev. 2010;2010(11):CD000025.
2. Webster LM, Conti-Ramsden F, Seed PT, Webb AJ, Nelson-Piercy C, Chappell LC. Impact of antihypertensive treatment on maternal and perinatal outcomes in pregnancy complicated by chronic hypertension: A systematic review and meta-analysis. J Am Heart Assoc. 2017;6(5):e005526.
3. Al Khalaf SY, O'Reilly ÉJ, Barrett PM, Leite DFB, Pawley LC, McCarthy FP, et al. Impact of chronic hypertension and antihypertensive treatment on adverse perinatal outcomes: Systematic review and meta-analysis. J Am Heart Assoc. 2021;10(9):e018494.

5.7 Hypertension in Chronic Kidney Disease

Sudhiranjan Dash Choudhury

INTRODUCTION

Chronic kidney disease (CKD) is defined as a condition which results in irreversible loss of renal function for ≥3 months. According to the recent guidelines, any one of them in presence of normal kidney function also can be included which are:
- Irreversible structural damage of the kidney or both the kidneys [as evidenced by imaging studies such as ultrasonography (USG), computed tomography (CT) scan, and magnetic resonance imaging (MRI), etc.].
- Renal histopathology suggestive of irreversible damage in spite of normal looking kidneys on imaging.
- Proteinuria more than normal values for >3 months.

Chronic kidney disease can be staged from 1 to 5 stages (Fig. 1).
Chronic kidney disease has been associated most often with hypertension. The pathogenesis of hypertension seems to be multifactorial. Hence to achieve the control of blood pressure (BP), the knowledge and mechanism of hypertension should be known to the treating physician. It is imperative that a multipronged approach will be required to get a target effect. It has been seen in different trials and evidence-based studies that CKD population benefit from tight control of BP not only to delay the progression of disease but also it resulted in improvement in hard endpoints such as cardiovascular and cerebrovascular morbidity and mortality. Meeting the requirement for tight BP control is never easy and to achieve that we require various tools such as active participation of patient in changing the lifestyle from sedentary to active, regular exercise, good dietary habit changes such as low salt intake, decreased consumption of saturated fat and refined sugar, increased consumption of roughage, weight reduction, and quitting smoking. Besides an intervention is required most often with drugs to control BP and blood sugar.

PATHOGENESIS OF HYPERTENSION IN CHRONIC KIDNEY DISEASE POPULATION

Renin-angiotensin-aldosterone system (RAAS) has been identified as one of the driver for hypertension genesis in many scientific studies. However, it has to be emphasized that this is not the only mechanism which can be attributable toward the development of hypertension.

GFR and ACR categories and risk of adverse outcomes		ACR categories (mg/mmol), description and range		
		<3 Normal to mildly increased	3–30 Moderately increased	>30 Severely increased
		A1	A2	A3
≥90 Normal or high	G1	No CKD in the absence of markers of kindly damage		
60–89 Mild reduction related to normal range for a young adult	G2			
45–59 Mild to moderate reduction	G3a¹			
30–44 Moderate to severe reduction	G3b			
15–29 Severe reduction	G4			
<15 Kidney failure	G5			

GFR categories (mL/min/1.73 m²), description and range

Increasing risk →

¹Consider using eGFR cystatin C for people with CKD G3aA1

FIG. 1: Classification of chronic kidney disease using glomerular filtration rate (GFR) and albumin-to-creatinine ratio (ACR) categories.

(ACR: albumin: creatinine ratio; CKD: chronic kidney disease; GFR: glomerular filtration rate)

Source: Adapted with permission from kidney disease: improving global outcomes (KDIGO) CKD work group (2013) KDIGO 2012 clinical practice guideline for the avaluation and management of chronic kidney disease. Kidney international (suppl. 3): 1–150.

Activation of various pathways in CKD population shown above ultimately results in increased extracellular volume and high total peripheral resistance.

Here we have to identify which mechanism is upregulated in these cobweb of interactions accordingly the management plan to be tailor-made for that patient. A one-glove-fit-all approach usually results in suboptimal control of BP resulting in the abovementioned complications and target organ damage which has to be avoided at any cost.

An in-depth knowledge of the above mechanisms is to be studied, for example: RAAS axis activation is more common in Caucasians with CKD. Hence, it is always beneficial to use either angiotensin-converting-enzyme (ACE) inhibitors and/or angiotensin-receptor blockers (ARBs) in those group of patients to achieve optimum result. Whereas in African Americans, RAAS activation is to the minimum rather increased sympathetic activity and salt retention resulting volume expansion are major causes of hypertension. Hence, rationally using diuretics with other agents will work better in controlling the BP rather than use of RAAS blockers alone. Likewise at different stages of CKD, different mechanisms play major roles. For example, in patients with CKD stage 4 onward, salt and water retention resulting in expanded extracellular fluid (ECF) volume are major drivers for hypertension contrary to in lesser CKD stages, RAAS mediators are more important. Also there are locally produced hormones indicative of endothelial dysfunction with various interaction results in hypertension in CKD populations. The major influencing factors which contribute toward hypertension will be described in the following paragraphs.

NITRIC OXIDE AND ENDOTHELIN

Nitric oxide (NO) is a potent vasodilator and endothelin-1 (ET-1) is a potent vasoconstrictor. To maintain the tone of the artery, a balance between NO production and ET-1 is essential. These are the local hormones produced from the endothelium which results in maintaining the tone of arteries and arterioles by smooth muscle contraction. Any disbalance in reduction of NO and increased production of ET-1 will result in potent vasoconstriction and the outcome being systemic hypertension. In different stages of CKD, endothelial disregulation sets in. Overproduction of reactive oxygen species (ROS) produces free oxygen radicals which reduce the NO by reducing super oxide dismutase (SOD) which produces free oxygen radical scavengers. Also, NO production reduces due to inhibition of nitric oxide synthase (NOS) enzyme. The entire above phenomenon gets exaggerated in CKD population resulting in hypertension.

ASYMMETRICAL DIMETHYLARGININE

Another way by which NO production is hampered is due to increased asymmetrical dimethylarginine (ADMA) activity. ADMA is a strong inhibitor of NOS. In CKD, uremic toxins directly inhibit L-arginine synthesis, which is a natural substrate for production of NO from endothelium. Also, ADMA level increases due to less filtration in renal failure. Besides the dimethylarginine dimethylamine hydrolase (DDAH) enzyme which degrades ADMA, its production decreases due to oxidative stress and uremic environment. Ultimately, it affects the cardiovascular health of the patient.

ROLE OF ENDOGENOUS DIGITALIS-LIKE FACTORS IN HYPERTENSION IN CHRONIC KIDNEY DISEASE POPULATION

Sodium pump or sodium potassium adenosine triphosphatase (ATPase) are present ubiquitously on all cells of human body. It has been identified that Na^+-K^+ ATPase channels are responsible for regulation of vascular resistance and sodium handling by release of natriuretic peptides in the vasculatures of human being. For the past couple of decades, digitalis is identified with properties to inhibit this transporter and is used for treatment of congestive heart failure. Besides a dysregulation of production of endogenous digitalis-like factor (EDLF) in circulation had been attributed for increased contractility of vascular smooth muscles resulting in increased vascular resistance. EDLF excretion gets impaired due to decline in glomerular filtration rate (GFR) in CKD which is responsible for intravascular volume expansion due to salt and water retention and increased peripheral resistance resulting in hypertension. This phenomenon is more applicable at later stages of CKD in CKD-stage 4 and CKD-stage 5 population or population on dialysis. Effective dialysis with ultrafiltration and salt restricted diet enhances the EDLF excretion and control of hypertension in this subset of population contrary to the belief of RAAS-mediated hypertension in CKD.

MANAGEMENT OF HYPERTENSION IN CHRONIC KIDNEY DISEASE POPULATION

The symptoms and signs and investigations pertaining to hypertension in CKD population are beyond the scope of this chapter and have been described elsewhere. However, salient points of management of this subset of population. I am describing in this chapter.

The management of hypertension can be grouped into two broad categories, i.e.:
1. Pre-end-stage renal disease (ESRD) population, i.e., CKD stage: 1 to 5.
2. ESRD population, i.e., CKD stage 5D.

Let us discuss the management of hypertension in CKD population.

Pre-end-stage Renal Disease Population, i.e., Chronic Kidney Disease Stage: 1 to 5

Hypertension in the predialysis population is most often due to RAAS-mediated hypertension. Also proteinuria and increased intraglomerular pressure due to loss of nephrons result in further progression of renal disease independent of etiology. Angiotensin-II, the final product of RAAS activation, is a strong vasoconstrictor responsible for production of not only intraglomerular hypertension but also a hormone which produces profibrotic cytokines such as transforming growth factor (TGF)-beta.

The above factor induces fibrogenesis and leads to glomerular sclerosis and interstitial fibrosis which are independent factors for progression of kidney disease. Besides angiotensin II is a potent stimulator for aldosterone which in return is responsible for increased sympathetic overactivity and salt and water retention which in return cause hypertension. The Pathway-2 study showed spironolactone as an effective "ADD-ON" medication for resistant hypertension. The only major side effect attributed being more frequent occurrences of hyperkalemia in subset of patients with renal failure. Recently done AMBER trial with use of patiromer and potassium binder showed promise in reducing these subset patients with hyperkalemia in bringing down the serum potassium to normal level. Hence, it is imperative in pre-ESRD patient's addition of ACE inhibitors or ARBs to block the RAAS will benefit the patient. However, as the patient progresses toward higher CKD stages, there will be a combination of volume excess and RAAS activation. Hence, addition of diuretics to control the salt and water also would be important. While doing so we have to closely watch the volume status and the estimated glomerular filtration rate (eGFR). In presence of volume depletion, the RAAS blockade can potentially tip the patient toward decrease in GFR due to low afferent arterial flow and vasodilatation of the efferent arteriole. Hence, a close watch on volume status and eGFR assessment is essential to do at intervals. Also, we have to closely watch for the hyperkalemia. If the serum creatinine change happens >20% from baseline level with hyperkalemia, then it is advisable to lower the doses of ACE inhibitors or ARBs or stop the medications temporarily. It is recommended to watch the serum creatinine and serum potassium initially after 2 weeks and once a week thereafter for 2 weeks to watch potential toxicity of this group of drugs. Potency wise both ACE inhibitors and ARBs can be used; however, the deciding factor would be cautiously watching the side effect profile of each category.

Hypertension Control in Chronic Kidney Disease Stage-5D Population

For those group of patients who are on dialysis, the hypertension control is little bit different as most often hypertension happens due to salt and water retention. Hence, in this group of patients, use of RAAS blockade has limited value. Whereas suggesting salt and water restriction with good effective dialysis will control the BP with minimum drugs. Frequent nocturnal hemodialysis (FHN) group study revealed almost minimal requirement of antihypertensive agents against conventional three times a week maintenance hemodialysis patients. Besides salt and water management, it was proposed that clearance of substances such as ADMA and DLI and others in dialysis could be the possible ways which result in better control of BP in those subset of patients. In a small subset of patients on dialysis, RAAS-mediated hypertension still could be prevalent. Identifying those will be essential as they respond well to RAAS blockade. Most often those group of patients will have intradialytic hypertension and a small addition of ACE inhibitor or ARBs will result in effective control of BP.

The target BP level to achieve in dialysis population is still controversial. However, with several literature and meta-analysis in hand, there was a consensus among nephrologist to keep the BP of 140-150 mm Hg systolic and 70-80 mm Hg diastolic predialysis should be achieved to reduce target organ damage.

A good control of BP when achieved in CKD population will not only reduce the cardiovascular and cerebrovascular mortality and morbidity, but also delay the progression of CKD. We have remembered most often it is difficult to achieve with one drug alone. We might have to aim at use of more than one drug with synergistic and additive effect to achieve the target goal.

SUMMARY

- CKD is irreversible loss of renal function for ≥3 months.
- According to recent guidelines, irreversible radiological structural damage of the kidney/renal histopathology suggestive of irreversible damage/proteinuria more than normal values for more than 3 months with normal renal functions.
- RAAS activation increased sympathetic activity and salt retention resulting volume expansion are major causes of hypertension.
- NO production is reduced by free oxygen radicals which reduce the NO by reducing super oxide dismutase (SOD) and due to increased ADMA (strong inhibitor of NOS).
- Hypertension in the predialysis population is most often due to RAAS-mediated hypertension. ACE inhibitors and ARBs with addition of diuretics (aldosterone antagonist) as the stage progresses are the standard line of management.
- In ESRD, use of RAAS blockade has limited value.
- Besides salt and water management, the clearance of substances such as ADMA and DLI and others in dialysis could be the possible reason.

MULTIPLE CHOICE QUESTIONS

1. CKD can be diagnosed in patients with normal kidney function by presence of one of the following, except:
    A. Irreversible structural damage of the kidney as evidenced on USG
    B. Presence of occult blood and epithelial cells in urine routine for consecutive 6 months
    C. Histopathology suggestive of irreversible damage
    D. Proteinuria more than normal values for more than 3 months

2. Pathogenesis of HTN in CKD includes the following:
    A. Increased sympathetic activity
    B. Salt and water retention
    C. RAAS system
    D. All of the above

3. The tone of artery and arterioles is maintained by:
    A. Vasodilation by nitric oxide
    B. Vasoconstriction by endothelin-1

C. Both fo them
D. None of the above

4. Routine investigations in CKD patients on ARB/ACE inhibitors include:
   A. Serum creatinine
   B. Serum electrolytes
   C. Urine routine
   D. All of the above

5. Angiotensin-II in CKD is responsible for the following pathogenesis:
   A. Intraglomerular hypertension
   B. Glomerular sclerosis
   C. Interstitial fibrosis
   D. All of the above

Answers

1—B   2—D   3—C   4—D   5—D

SUGGESTED READINGS

1. Fu EL, Clase CM, Evans M, Lindholm B, Rotmans JI, Dekker FW, et al. Comparative effectiveness of renin-angiotensin system inhibitors and calcium channel blockers in individuals with advanced CKD: A nationwide observational cohort study. Am J Kidney Dis. 2021;77(5):719-29.e1.
2. Hundemer GL, Knoll GA, Petrcich W, Hiremath S, Ruzicka M, Burns KD, et al. Kidney, cardiac, and safety outcomes associated with α-blockers in patients with CKD: A population-based cohort study. Am J Kidney Dis. 2021;77(2):178-89.e1.
3. Barcellos FC, Del Vecchio FB, Reges A, Mielke G, Santos IS, Umpierre D, et al. Exercise in patients with hypertension and chronic kidney disease: a randomized controlled trial. J Hum Hypertens. 2018;32(6):397-407.
4. Meuleman Y, Hoekstra T, Dekker FW, Navis G, Vogt L, van der Boog PJM, et al. Sodium restriction in patients with CKD: A randomized controlled trial of self-management support. Am J Kidney Dis. 2017;69(5):576-86.
5. Galbraith L, Jacobs C, Hemmelgarn BR, Donald M, Manns BJ, Jun M. Chronic disease management interventions for people with chronic kidney disease in primary care: a systematic review and meta-analysis. Nephrol Dial Transplant. 2018;33(1):112-21.
6. Chung EY, Ruospo M, Natale P, Bolignano D, Navaneethan SD, Palmer SC, et al. Aldosterone antagonists in addition to renin angiotensin system antagonists for preventing the progression of chronic kidney disease. Cochrane Database Syst Rev. 2020;10(10):CD007004.

5.8 Perioperative Hypertension

Shivani Kamat

INTRODUCTION

Perioperative *hypertension is defined as* elevation *of blood pressure above the* target range in patients with and without pre-existing *hypertension during the preoperative, intraoperative, and postoperative periods.*[1]
The perioperative period can be *divided into three* stages.[2]
1. *Preoperative*: The period *from patient admission* in the hospital to the start of the surgery.
2. *Intraoperative*: The period in *between the transfer of patient to* operation room till *end of surgery.*
3. *Postoperative*: *This period* lasts from end of surgery up to 48-72 hours postsurgery.

About 5-35% of patients are likely to undergo acute elevation in blood pressure during the perioperative period which results in increase in probability of complications and *mortality* rate which rises by four-fold.[3] The perioperative complications in hypertensive patients usually include cardiovascular, cerebrovascular, and renovascular pathologies along with increase in bleeding rate.[3] A study in patients with isolated systolic hypertension has shown 30% increase in unfavorable outcomes in those undergoing cardiac surgery.[4]

In general, the risk of complications is directly proportional to rise in blood pressure. Thus, before start of any operation, it is important to determine predictors of high blood pressure in order to adequately control it. For example, a study conducted demonstrates increased pulse rate *to be an independent risk factor for* postoperative neurological *complications* and *cardiac* failure.[5] Another study conducted in patients undergoing endarterectomy found that hypertension or hypotension during the postoperative period in which intravenous (IV) *administration of vasoactive drugs* was needed, is associated with increased risk of morbidity and mortality in the 1 year period following the operation.[6] Thus, stressing importance of continuous blood pressure monitoring in perioperative patients. Intraoperative high blood pressure is also associated with extended duration of hospital stay and increased mortality rate. However, intraoperative blood pressure fluctuations due to anesthesia are largely influenced by preoperative baseline blood pressure of an individual as the study conducted by Prys-Robert et al. demonstrated that patients with normal blood pressure and well-controlled hypertensives reacted to anesthesia in the same manner while those with poorly controlled blood pressure showed fluctuations with sudden drop at the start of anesthesia followed by elevated blood pressure at the end as a result of alteration in vascular resistance.[2] Thus, perioperative hypertension can largely *be avoided* if *the blood pressure is* adequately *controlled* in *the* preoperative period by optimal medical management.

ETIOLOGY OF PERIOPERATIVE HYPERTENSION

Causes for perioperative hypertension are as follows:[7]
- Poorly controlled pre-existing essential hypertension
- Over administration of IV vasopressor
- Excessive intraoperative fluid therapy
- Mobilization of fluid from the extravascular space in the postoperative period
- Anesthesia induction
- Airway instrumentation
- During the intraoperative/early postoperative period, blood pressure increases *due to sympathetic stimulation* which occurs *as a result of* hypothermia, hypoxia, or bladder distension
- Sudden withdrawal of long-term angiotensin-receptor blocker (ARB)/angiotensin-converting enzyme inhibitor (ACEI) prior to surgery
- Alcohol withdrawal and use of cocaine
- Anxiety and pain

PERIOPERATIVE EVALUATION FOR HYPERTENSIVE PATIENTS

In hypertensive patients, precautions should be taken before administration of general anesthesia and the preoperative evaluation in terms of personal and medication history, addiction history, baseline blood pressure readings, antihypertensive medicines, dosages, comorbidities, and hypertension-mediated end-organ damage is as follows:

Preoperative Evaluation
- Should be done at least 1 week prior to surgery
- Thorough history of the patient including use of recreational drugs substance
- Measuring blood pressure at timely interval
- Adequacy of blood pressure control
- Assessment of antihypertensive medications
- Modification in dosages
- Determining change in antihypertensive medication with respect to drug class and single or combination pills
- Assessment for end-organ damage

If a patient has been diagnosed as a hypertensive in the preoperative period, it is necessary to verify if its white-coat hypertension or sustained, primary or secondary hypertension as this distinction will direct the management.

Intraoperative Evaluation

Induction and maintenance of anesthesia—before start of an operation, an anesthesiologist should be aware of the patient history, baseline blood pressure, and heart rate and previous reaction to anesthesia and medicine allergy.
- Close *monitoring of vital signs*: *Blood pressure, heart rate, respiratory rate, and* oxygen saturation
- Blood pressure monitoring with an invasive transducing method
- Blood pressure monitoring every 5 minutes using noninvasive cuff method[6]
- Monitoring for complications in high-risk patients
- Anticipation of hypotension to anesthetic drugs
- Close monitoring of vasopressor and fluid administration
- Limit duration of direct laryngoscopy and endotracheal intubation

Postoperative Evaluation

Anticipation of acute postoperative hypertension between the first 20 minutes and 4 hours postsurgery is crucial as untreated postoperative hypertension *can lead to increased risk of* cardiovascular, neurological, and *surgical site* complications.[8]
- Monitoring for orthostatic hypotension
- Anticipation of fluid overload
- Continuous blood pressure monitoring and management especially in the first 4 hours postsurgery
- Evaluation of end-organ function
- Additional care in *cardiothoracic, vascular, head and neck, and* neurological surgical *procedures is* recommended.

PERIOPERATIVE BLOOD PRESSURE MANAGEMENT

The aim of perioperative pharmacotherapy is rapid and safe reduction in blood pressure without causing organ hypoperfusion. The commonly used drugs are as follows **(Table 1)**:

TABLE 1: Summary of commonly used drugs.

Drug	Class	Dose	Onset and duration of action
Labetalol	Combined α + β-blocker	*Loading dose*: 20 mg followed by 20–80 mg incremental dose every 10 minutes Alternatively, infusion 1–2 mg/min after initial loading dose until hypotensive effect	Onset 2–5 minutes; reaches peak at 5–15 minutes, lasts up to 4 hours; elimination half-life 5.5 hours

Continued

Continued

Drug	Class	Dose	Onset and duration of action
Esmolol	β-blocker	Loading dose 500–1,000 µg/kg in 1 minute, then infusion starting at 50 µg/kg/min increasing up to 300 µg/kg/min as required	Rapid onset 60 seconds; short duration of action 10–20 minutes
Enalaprilat	ACE inhibitor	1.25 mg over 5 minutes every 6 hours increased by 1.25 mg at 12–24 hours to a maximum 5 mg every 6 hours	Variable response, slow-onset, and long duration of action, titration difficult
Fenoldopam	Peripheral dopamine-1 (DA) receptor agonist	Starting dose 0.1 µg/kg/min, increasing by 0.05–0.1 µg/kg/min up to a maximum 1.6 µg/kg/min	Onset within 5 minutes, maximal response by 15 minutes, duration of action 30–60 minutes, elimination half-life 5 minutes
Hydralazine	Direct-acting arteriolar Vasodilator	• IV bolus: 10–20 mg every 1–4 hours as required • IV infusion: Loading dose 0.1 mg/kg followed by continuous infusion 1.5–5 µg/kg/min	Onset 5–15 minutes, circulating half-life 3 hours, fall in BP may last up to 12 hours
Nicardipine	Dihydropyridine CCB – second generation	5 mg/h, incrementing by 2.5 mg/h every 5–15 minutes not to exceed 15 mg/h	Onset 5–15 minutes, duration of action 4–6 hours
Nitroglycerin	Arterial and venous dilator	Starting infusion at 5 µg/min, increased by 5 µg/min every 3–5 minutes up to 20 µg/min	Onset 2–5 minutes, duration of action 10–20 minutes
Nitroprusside	Arterial and venous dilator	Initial infusion 0.25–0.3 µg/kg/min, increase by 0.5 µg/kg/min every 1–2 minutes to achieve desired results	Rapid onset in seconds, duration of action 1–2 minutes, plasma half-life 3–4 minutes

(BP: blood pressure; CCB: calcium channel blocker; IV: intravenous)

Esmolol

- Ultra-short-acting cardioselective, β-adrenergic blocking agent
- Metabolism of esmolol is via rapid hydrolysis of ester linkages by red blood cell (RBC) esterases and is not dependent on renal or hepatic function.

- Decreases atrial pressure by decreasing heart rate and myocardial contractility and thus cardiac output
- 500–1,000 µg/kg loading dose over 1 minute, followed by an infusion starting at 50 µg/kg/min and increasing up to 300 µg/kg/min
- Rapid onset (60 seconds) and short duration of action (10–20 minutes)
- Anemia will prolong its "short half-life."

Caution

Chronic obstructive lung disease—bronchospasm

Labetalol

- Selective α1-adrenergic receptor blocker and nonselective β-adrenergic blocker
- Metabolized by the liver to an inactive glucuronide conjugate
- Pregnancy-induced hypertensive crisis.
- Hypotensive effect of labetalol begins within 2–5 minutes after its IV administration
- *Onset of action*: 2–5 minutes reaching a peak: 5–15 minutes and duration of action—2–4 hours
- Elimination half-life of labetalol is approximately 5.5 hours.
- *Administration*: At a loading dose of 20 mg, incremental doses of 20–80 mg at repeated 10-minute intervals until the desired blood pressure is achieved.
  Or
- Initial loading dose, an infusion commencing at 1–2 mg/min and titrated up to until the desired hypotensive effect is achieved is particularly effective.

Caution

Heart failure and severe sinus bradycardia/heart block greater than first degree and asthma.

Nitroglycerin

- Direct vasodilator of peripheral capacitance and resistance vessels
- Decreases preload hence decreases left ventricular end-diastolic volume and pressure, and reduces myocardial oxygen demand
- Dilates coronary arteries, increasing the blood supply to ischemic regions of the heart
- *Time of onset*: 2–5 minutes, duration of action approximately 10–20 minutes
- Eliminated by hepatic metabolism approximately 1–4 minutes

Sodium Nitroprusside

- *Arterial and venous vasodilator*: Decreasing both afterload and preload
- Decrease in peripheral resistance
- Drug of choice for hypertensive emergencies, immediate onset of action, and duration of effect of only 2 minutes

- Onset of action of seconds, duration of action of 1–2 minutes, and a plasma half-life of 3–4 minutes
- *Caution*: In patients with hypertensive encephalopathy or following a cerebrovascular accident.
- Accumulation of cyanide and thiocyanate (eliminated through the kidneys)
- Patients can develop cyanide toxicity as early as 6–8 hours after initiation of the infusion.
- *Tachyphylaxis*: Occurs in high infusion rates (>3 µg/kg/min) and prolonged administration (>72 hours)
- Initial starting dose of 0.5 µg/kg/min; titrate as tolerated. The duration of treatment should be as short as possible and the infusion rate should not be >2 µg/kg/min.

SUMMARY

- Perioperative hypertension is defined as elevated blood pressure during the pre-, intra-, and postoperative period lasting from admission of patient in the hospital up to 48–72 hours postsurgery.
- Surgical stress is a common phenomenon which contributes to sympathetic, metabolic, and hematological changes. However, exaggerated blood pressure response is negatively associated with postoperative complications including cardiovascular and renal events as well as stroke.
- The most common cause of preoperative and intraoperative hypertension is poorly controlled pre-existing essential hypertension and fluid overload is the common reason for postoperative hypertension.
- Perioperative hypertension evaluation is of utmost importance as it can also lead to diagnosis of long-standing undiagnosed high blood pressure.
- Pharmacotherapy in perioperative hypertension should be directed toward rapid and safe blood pressure reduction and prevention of end-organ hypoperfusion.
- New agents such as fenoldopam, nicardipine, and clevidipine are valuable additions to the enalaprilat, labetalol, nitroglycerin, esmolol, and hydralazine which are other effective pharmacological options.
- Sodium nitroprusside is to be used only when other IV antihypertensive agents are not available.

MULTIPLE CHOICE QUESTIONS

1. Causes of perioperative hypertension includes the following:
   A. Sympathetic stimulation due to pain
   B. Airway instrumentation
   C. Induction of anesthesia
   D. All of the above

2. Metabolism of esmolol is dependent on:
   A. Rapid hydrolysis of ester linkages by RBC esterase
   B. Renal excretion
   C. Hepatic excretion
   D. All of the above

3. Action of nitroglycerin includes the following:
   A. Reduces myocardial oxygen demand
   B. Decreases left ventricular end-diastolic volume
   C. Dilates coronary arteries
   D. All of the above

4. Which of the following is a false statement?
   A. Sodium nitroprusside is an arterial vasodilator
   B. Sodium nitroprusside is a venous vasodilator
   C. Sodium nitroprusside increases preload
   D. Sodium nitroprusside decreases peripheral resistance

5. Which of the following is a false statement?
   A. Labetalol is a selective alpha-1 adrenergic receptor blocker
   B. Labetalol is a selective beta-adrenergic receptor blocker
   C. Labetalol is metabolized by the liver
   D. Labetalol is metabolized to an inactive glucuronide conjugate

Answers

1—D   2—A   3—D   4—C   5—B

REFERENCES

1. Prys-Roberts C, Greene LT, Meloche R, Foëx P. Studies of anaesthesia in relation to hypertension. II. Haemodynamic consequences of induction and endotracheal intubation. Br J Anaesth. 1971;43(6):531-47.
2. Meng L, Yu W, Wang T, Zhang L, Heerdt PM, Gelb AW. Blood pressure targets in perioperative care. Provisional considerations based on a comprehensive literature review. 2018;72(4):806-17.
3. Kar G. Perioperative management of hypertension. [online] Available from: https://apiindia.org/uploads/pdf/progress_in_medicine_2017/mu_50.pdf. [Last accessed December, 2022].
4. HaAronson S, Boisvert D, Lapp W. Isolated systolic hypertension is associated with adverse outcomes fromcoronary artery bypass grafting surgery. Anaesth Analog. 2002;94(5):1079-84.
5. Fontes ML, Aronson S, Mathew JP, Miao Y, Drenger B, Barash PG, et al. Pulse pressure and risk of adverse outcome in coronary bypass surgery. Anesth Analg. 2008;107(4):1122-29.
6. Link A, Selejan S, Walenta K, Reil JC, Böhm M. Therapie des peri- und postoperativen hypertensiven Notfalls [Treatment of peri- and postoperative hypertensive emergencies]. Dtsch Med Wochenschr. 2009;134(14):701-7.

7. Mohseni S, Behnam-Roudsari S, Tarbiat M, Shaker P, Shivaie S, Shafiee MA. Perioperative hypertension etiologies in patients undergoing noncardiac surgery in University Health Network Hospitals–Canada from 2015–2020. Integr Blood Press Control. 2022;15:23-32.
8. Viljoen JF, Estafanous FG, Tarazi RC. Acute hypertension immediately after coronary artery surgery. J Thorac Cardiovasc Surg. 1976;71(4):548-50.

SUGGESTED READINGS

1. Aronson S, Dyke CM, Stierer KA, Levy JH, Cheung AT, Lumb PD, et al. The ECLIPSE trials: comparative studies of clevidipine to nitroglycerin, sodium nitroprusside, and nicardipine for acute hypertension treatment in cardiac surgery patients. Anesth Analg. 2008;107(4):1110-21.
2. Villarreal EG, Flores S, Kriz C, Iranpour N, Bronicki RA, Loomba RS. Sodium nitroprusside versus nicardipine for hypertension management after surgery: A systematic review and meta-analysis. J Card Surg. 2020;35(5):1021-28.
3. Aronson S. Clevidipine in the treatment of perioperative hypertension: assessing safety events in the ECLIPSE trials. Expert Rev CardiovascTher. 2009;7(5):465-72.
4. Gill R, Goldstein S. Evaluation and management of perioperative hypertension. 2022.
5. Halpern NA, Goldberg M, Neely C, Sladen RN, Goldberg JS, Floyd J, et al. Postoperative hypertension: a multicenter, prospective, randomized comparison between intravenous nicardipine and sodium nitroprusside. Crit Care Med. 1992;20(12):1637-43.

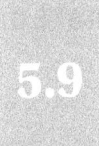

Hypertension in Special Subsets: Ischemic Heart Disease

Ruchit Shah, Nandhakumar Vasu

INTRODUCTION

European Society of Cardiology (ESC) 2018 guidelines defined systemic hypertension (SHT) as office or home systolic blood pressure (SBP) ≥140 mm Hg and/or diastolic blood pressure (DBP) ≥90 mm Hg and isolated systolic hypertension is defined as SBP ≥140 mm Hg and DBP <90 mm Hg.

The understanding of genesis of IHD continues to evolve with the identification of inflammatory elements and genetic risk factors. Vasoconstrictor hormones, cytokines as well as various inflammatory mediators promote leukocyte adhesion to endothelial wall surface, which is the inciting event in the pathophysiology of IHD.

The cardiovascular (CV) risk rises with the stage of hypertension and the risk escalates exponentially with additional risk factors. Hypertension-mediated target organ damage escalates the risk still further. Ischemic heart disease (IHD) is the most common type of target-organ damage. IHD may be associated with adverse outcomes such as myocardial infarction (MI), heart failure, ventricular arrhythmias, and sudden cardiac death. The INTERHEART study showed that ~25% of the population-attributable risk of a MI can be accounted by SHT. Because of successful efforts of developed countries to lower SBP, there has been a decline in IHD mortality. The prevalence of SHT remains very high and age remains as its strongest risk factor.

PREVALENCE OF ISCHEMIC HEART DISEASE (TABLE 1)

TABLE 1: Prevalence of ischemic heart disease.

Age group	Prevalence
18–39 years	7.3%
40–59 years	32.4%
>60 years	65%

CARDIOVASCULAR RISK ESTIMATION IN HYPERTENSIVE PATIENTS

The patient's CV risk can be estimated from the American College of Cardiology/American Heart Association (ACC/AHA) risk estimator or the SCORE system.

SYSTEMATIC CORONARY RISK EVALUATION SYSTEM—10-YEAR CARDIOVASCULAR RISK CATEGORIES (TABLE 2)

TABLE 2: Systematic coronary risk evaluation system—10-year cardiovascular risk categories.[1-3]

Low risk	Moderate risk	High risk	Very high risk
10 years SCORE of <1%	10 years SCORE of ≥1 to< 5%	10 years SCORE of 5–10%	10 years SCORE of ≥10%
	Grade 2 SHT	Hypertensive LVH	Clinical CVD—MI, coronary revascularization, stroke, TIA, aortic aneurysm, and PAD
		eGFR 30–59 mL/min/ 1.73 m²	Significant plaque ≥50% stenosis by angiography or ultrasound
		Total cholesterol >310 mg/dL	eGFR 30 mL/min/1.73 m²
		Grade 3 SHT or DM	DM with target organ damage

(CVD: cardiovascular disease; DM: diabetes mellitus; eGFR: estimated glomerular filtration rate; LVH: left ventricular hypertrophy; MI: myocardial infarction; PAD: peripheral arterial disease; SHT: systemic hypertension; TIA: transient ischemic attack)

PROGNOSTIC RISK FACTORS IN HYPERTENSIVE PATIENTS (TABLE 3)

TABLE 3: Prognostic risk factors in hypertensive patients.[1,3,7,8]

Risk factors for cardiovascular diseases	Subclinical hypertension-mediated organ damage	Established target organ damage
Age >55 years (M); >65 years (F)	Left ventricular hypertrophy (LVH)—by echocardiography (ECG)	Cerebrovascular disease – Ischemic or hemorrhagic stroke, transient ischemic attack
Systolic, diastolic BP, and pulse pressure	Ankle brachial index <0.9	Cardiovascular disease: hypertensive heart disease, LVH, left atrial enlargement, atrial fibrillation, coronary artery disease, myocardial infarction, heart failure with preserved ejection fraction, and heart failure with reduced ejection fraction
Smoking	Microalbuminuria	Renovascular or renal parenchymal disease

Continued

Continued

Risk factors for cardiovascular diseases	Subclinical hypertension-mediated organ damage	Established target organ damage
Dyslipidemia (LDL-C >115 mg/dL)	eGFR <60 mL/min/1.73 m^2	Peripheral arterial disease
Diabetes	Carotid wall thickening	Retinopathy
Obesity		
Family history of premature cardiovascular disease		
Sedentary lifestyle		
Early menopause		
Psychological and socioeconomic factors		
Resting heart rate >80 bpm		

(BP: blood pressure; eGFR: estimated glomerular filtration rate; LDL-C: low-density lipoprotein cholesterol)

PREVENTION OF ISCHEMIC HEART DISEASE IN SYSTEMIC HYPERTENSION

Identifying these factors and treating or preventing will help in the prevention of IHD. Active search for asymptomatic hypertension-mediated target organ damage (HMOD) by looking for left ventricular hypertrophy in electrocardiogram (ECG) or echocardiogram (ECHO) or evidence of arterial stiffening like increased pulse pressure and aggressive treatment of SHT may prevent IHD. High DBP is associated with increased IHD risk and is more commonly elevated in younger (<50 years) versus older patients. Beyond midlife as a consequence of arterial stiffening SBP assumes even greater importance as a risk factor. A consistent and significant SBP difference of >15 mm Hg between arms is associated with an elevated IHD risk. Treatment of SHT-induced regression of left ventricular hypertrophy (LVH) by ECG or ECHO is associated with a reduction in IHD risk. Every 10 mm Hg reduction in SBP by antihypertensive therapy reduces the incidence of IHD by 17%.

DYSLIPIDEMIA

Management of concomitant CV risk in patients with IHD and hypertension is important. Atherogenic dyslipidemia is one among the important risk factor. Dyslipidemia in the form of elevated triglycerides and low-density lipoprotein-cholesterol (LDL-C) and low high-density lipoprotein (HDL) cholesterol when present along with SHT increases the CV risk. The benefit of adding a statin to antihypertensive therapy in patients without previous CV events has been demonstrated in Justification for the Use of statins in Prevention: an Intervention Trial Evaluating Rosuvastatin (JUPITER) and Heart Outcomes Prevention Evaluation-3 (HOPE-3) trials. The LDL-C lowering to <130 mg/dL reduced the incidence of CV events by 44% and 24% respectively in JUPITER and HOPE-3 trials. Hence, use of statins in hypertensive individuals with moderate-to-high risk is justifiable. When established IHD is present and the CV risk is very high, statins should be given with aim of reducing LDL-C to <70 mg/dL or a reduction of ≥50% if the baseline LDL-C is between 70 and 135 mg/dL.

MANAGEMENT OF HYPERTENSION FOR SECONDARY PREVENTION OF CORONARY EVENTS

The cardioprotective effects arise from the control of blood pressure (BP) irrespective of the drug class.

Any of the first-line drugs may be used.

Dual renin–angiotensin–aldosterone system (RAAS) blockade [angiotensin-converting enzyme (ACE) inhibitors + angiotensin receptor blocker (ARB)] is not advisable.

MANAGEMENT OF HYPERTENSION IN ACUTE CORONARY SYNDROME

In acute coronary syndrome (ACS) patients, BP must be lowered with intravenous Nitroglycerin after giving intravenous metoprolol or esmolol to prevent reflex tachycardia. Beta-blockers must be used cautiously in patients with left ventricular dysfunction or heart failure. Nitroprusside can cause coronary steal and must be avoided. Hypotension must be avoided.

MANAGEMENT OF HYPERTENSION IN ESTABLISHED ISCHEMIC HEART DISEASE (TABLE 4)

In patients with stable coronary artery disease (CAD) and SHT, those who were treated with antihypertensive therapy with the target of SBP ≥140 mm Hg and a DBP ≥80 mm Hg were associated with increased risk of CV events. A much lower target of SBP <120 mm Hg and DBP <70 mm Hg was also associated with increased CV events. This is the J-curve phenomenon. The existence of J-curve phenomenon in CAD patients whether persists after revascularization remains questionable.

TABLE 4: Systemic hypertension (SHT) with established ischemic heart disease (IHD)[2,6]

SBP	120–129 mm Hg
DBP	70–79 mm Hg
Age ≥65 years SBP	130–139 mm Hg
Age ≥65 years DBP	70–79 mm Hg
SHT with post-MI	Renin–angiotensin–aldosterone system blockers (ACE inhibitors or ARB) and beta-blockers (single combination pill)

Continued

Continued

SHT with stable angina	Beta-blockers and calcium channel blockers
	ACE inhibitors, ARB or thiazide diuretics may be added

(ACE: angiotensin-converting enzyme; ARB: angiotensin receptor blocker; DBP: diastolic blood pressure; MI: myocardial infarction; SBP: systolic blood pressure)

SALIENT FEATURES

- 25% of the population attributable risk of MI can be accounted by SHT.
- Systematic Coronary Risk Evaluation (SCORE) system calculates the 10-year risk of a first fatal atherosclerotic event, in relation to age, sex, smoking habits, SBP, and total cholesterol level.
- SBP target of 130–139 mm Hg and DBP target of 70–79 mm Hg is recommended for prevention of IHD in SHT patients.
- In established IHD patients, a target BP of <130/80 mm Hg is recommended, but do not decrease below 120/70 mm Hg.
- In patients with high or very high risk, a reduction of LDL-C to 50% from the baseline is recommended to prevent fatal CV event with a target LDL-C <70 mg/dL.

SUMMARY

- IHD is the most common type of target-organ damage caused by hypertension.
- SCORE system gives a 10-year CV risk category.
- Prognostic factors include age, SBP/DBP/pulse pressure (PP), smoking, dyslipidemia, family history, diabetes, obesity, sedentary lifestyle, early menopause, psychological and socioeconomic factors.
- Active search for asymptomatic HMOD by looking for LVH in ECG or ECHO or evidence of arterial stiffening is important.
- When established IHD is present and the CV risk is very high, statins should be given with aim of reducing LDL-C to <70 mg/dL or a reduction of ≥50% if the baseline LDL-C is between 70 and 135 mg/dL.
- In ACS patients, BP must be lowered with intravenous Nitroglycerin after giving intravenous metoprolol or esmolol.
- In patients with stable CAD and SHT, a much lower target of SBP <120 mm Hg and DBP <70 mm Hg was also associated with increased CV events.

MULTIPLE CHOICE QUESTIONS

1. Risk factors for developing IHD are the following, except:
   A. SHT
   B. Smoking
   C. LVH
   D. Alcohol intake

2. ESC 2018 guidelines define isolated systolic hypertension as:
   A. SBP >160 mm Hg and DBP <90 mm Hg
   B. SBP >150 mm Hg and DBP <90 mm Hg
   C. SBP >140 mm Hg and DBP <90 mm Hg
   D. SBP >160 mm Hg and DBP <80 mm Hg

3. The resting heart rate above which it is a risk factor of developing IHD in SHT patients:
   A. >100
   B. >80
   C. >110
   D. >60

4. The recommended target of SBP in IHD is:
   A. <130 mm Hg but not <120 mm Hg
   B. <140 mm Hg but not <130 mm Hg
   C. <120 mm Hg
   D. <110 mm Hg

5. SCORE CV risk stratification—high risk indicate 10-year SCORE of:
   A. 5–10%
   B. 1–5%
   C. >10%
   D. >20%

Answers

1—D   2—C   3—B   4—A   5—A

REFERENCES

1. Yusuf S, Hawken S, Ounpuu S, Dans T, Avezum A, Lanas F, et al. Effect of potentially modifiable risk factors associated with myocardial infarction in 52 countries (the INTERHEART study): case control study. Lancet. 2004;364:937-52.
2. Williams B, Manica G, Spiering W, AgabitiRosei E, Azizi M, Burnier M, et al. 2018 ESC/ESH Guidelines for the management of arterial hypertension. Eur Heart J. 2018;39:3021-104.
3. Margolis KL, O'Connor PJ, Morgan TM, Buse JB, Cohen RM, Cushman WC, et al. Outcomes of combined cardiovascular risk factor management strategies in type 2 diabetes: the ACCORD randomizedtrial. Diabetes Care. 2014;37:1721-8.
4. Yusuf S, Bosch J, Dagenais G, Zhu J, Xavier D, Liu L, et al. Cholesterol lowering in intermediate-risk persons without cardiovascular disease. N Engl J Med. 2016;374:2021-31.
5. Vidal-Petiot E, Ford I, Greenlaw N, Ferrari R, Fox KM, Tardif JC, et al. Cardiovascular event rates and mortality according to achieved systolic and diastolic blood pressurein patients with stable coronary artery disease: an international cohort study. Lancet. 2016;388:2142-52.
6. Agbor-Etang BB, Setaro JF. Management of hypertension in patients with ischemic heart disease. Curr Cardiol Rep. 2015;17(12):119.

7. Kokubo Y, Matsumoto C. Hypertension is a risk factor for several types of heart disease: Review of prospective studies. Adv Exp Med Biol. 2017;956:419-26.
8. van Oort S, Beulens JWJ, van Ballegooijen AJ, Grobbee DE, Larsson SC. Association of cardiovascular risk factors and lifestyle behaviors with hypertension: A Mendelian Randomization Study. Hypertension. 2020;76()6:1971-9.

5.10 Management of Hypertension in Pulmonary Diseases

Nimish Shah

INTRODUCTION

The prevalence of hypertension in patients suffering from respiratory comorbidities is only increasing with increased longevity among patients as the incidence of coronary artery disease (CAD) also increases.

Hypertension, CAD, and diabetes are frequently encountered which may result as a side effect of the drugs used to treat or manage such patients.

For the ease of management, hypertension management can be discussed in obstructive airways disease (OAD) (asthma, chronic OAD, and bronchiectasis), and other respiratory conditions.

In patients with non-OAD, conditions such as pulmonary fibrosis, sarcoidosis, and other conditions, a majority of the patients may be on long-term steroids, which lead to hypertension and weight gain.

More commonly, difficulties and dilemmas arise in management of hypertension in asthma and COPD or poorly controlled bronchiectasis (OADs).

ANGIOTENSIN–CONVERTING ENZYME INHIBITORS

Angiotensin-converting enzyme inhibitors (ACEIs) are frequently associated with a dry cough as a side effect. This is not restricted to patients with underlying respiratory conditions only. The cough is generally dry in nature, irritant, and persistent. It is rarely productive. The etiology of the cough is due to bradykinin release. Important to note that the cough can present even if the patient has been on it for a substantial amount of time, and should be considered as a cause for a chronic cough. There has been limited evidence to show that ACEIs can aggravate symptoms of asthma, but case reports have been published regarding the same. One needs to exclude all other causes of exacerbation before considering switching of antihypertensives in a controlled hypertensive.

ANGIOTENSIN-RECEPTOR BLOCKERS

Angiotensin-receptor blockers (ARBs) do not have any reported contraindications in asthma or chronic obstructive pulmonary disease (COPD). Patients who develop a cough due to ACEI can be switched to ARBs safely.

BETA-BLOCKERS

In asthmatics, beta-blockers (BBs) can cause increased bronchial obstruction and airway reactivity, as well as resistance to the effects of inhaled or oral beta-receptor agonists. However, with newer and more selective drugs (metoprolol, atenolol, bisoprolol, nebivolol, and esmolol) added to the basket, one can consider using these in asthmatics with close monitoring. Systematic reviews and meta-analysis[1] on the acute clinical effects on pulmonary function show that β-1 selective blockers significantly reduced forced expiratory volume in the first second (FEV_1) by 7% and attenuated the bronchodilator response to inhaled beta-2-selective agonists by 10%.

Nonselective BBs had more profound effects on pulmonary function: FEV_1 was significantly reduced by 10%, and the bronchodilator response to inhaled beta-2-selective was reduced by 20%.

In older asthmatics, with mild symptoms, a cardioselective BB can be tried with supervision.

In summary, BBs are best avoided in asthma.

In COPD, many patients have concomitant conditions such as CAD (coexists in up to 27% of COPD patients that require the use of BBs). BBs are often avoided in these patients because of fear of bronchospasm and possible adverse reactions, despite the known cardiovascular mortality and morbidity benefit. This is mainly based on anecdotal evidence and case reports citing acute bronchospasm following the administration of BB. COPD patients are at greater risk of ischemic heart disease than asthmatics, so would benefit from the use of BBs. On the other hand, they also have more severe airway obstruction, so may be more sensitive to small changes in FEV_1 due to beta-blockade. Large meta-analyses were published by Salpeter et al., where randomized, blinded, placebo-controlled trials that studied the effects of cardioselective BBs on FEV_1, symptoms, and the use of inhaled β2-agonists in patients with reactive airway disease were selected, of which, there were 19 single-dose treatment studies and 10 continued treatment studies. The conclusion was that cardioselective BBs do not produce clinically significant adverse respiratory effects in patients with mild-to-moderate reactive airway disease, and that they should not be withheld from these patients.

Thus, in conclusion, BBs reduce mortality in patients with COPD and coexisting CAD and should be used whenever possible. Cardioselective BBs are safe in patients with COPD who have an indication for their use. Nonselective BBs are better avoided in general.

Recently, there has been interest in an additional group called ACOS (asthma chronic obstructive pulmonary disease overlap syndrome) with there is evidence of reversibility in a COPD phenotype. Although no guidelines have been published for BB in the same, once should use BB, especially nonselective, with caution and under supervision.

CALCIUM CHANNEL BLOCKERS

This group of drugs are the preferred choice for the treatment of hypertension in asthma. In addition to effectively lowering the blood pressure, they also have the theoretical advantages of opposing muscle contraction in tracheobronchial smooth muscle, inhibiting mast cell degranulation, and possibly reinforcing the bronchodilator effect of beta-agonists. One has to be cautious of fluid retention and constipation in older patients with amlodipine.

DIURETICS

Diuretics can be effectively used in OAD, but the potential for serious hypokalemia must be recognized. This problem is related to the ability of inhaled beta-2 receptor agonists to drive potassium into the cells and of oral corticosteroids to mildly enhance urinary potassium excretion. In COPD, patients who develop *cor pulmonale* do benefit with additional diuresis along with working as an antihypertensive.

SUMMARY OF RECOMMENDATIONS OF ANTIHYPERTENSIVES IN OAD (TABLE 1)

TABLE 1: Summary of recommendations of anti-hypertensives in obstructive airways disease.[1,2]

Class	Recommendation
ACEI	Safe, cough as side effect
ARB	Safe
Beta blockers	*Asthma*: Avoid *COPD*: Safe with caution *ACOS*: No recommendations, with caution
Calcium channel blockers	Safe, recommended choice
Diuretics	*Asthma*: Beware risk of hypokalemia *COPD*: Safe with same risk of hypokalemia

(ACEI: angiotensin-converting enzyme inhibitor; ACOS: asthma chronic obstructive pulmonary disease overlap syndrome; ARB: angiotensin receptor blocker; COPD: chronic obstructive pulmonary disease)

SUMMARY

- Difficulties and dilemmas arise in management of hypertension in asthma and COPD.
- There has been limited evidence to show that ACEIs can aggravate symptoms of asthma except dry cough.
- ARBs do not have any reported contraindications in asthma or COPD.
- In older asthmatics, with mild symptoms, a cardioselective BB can be tried with supervision; however, BBs are best avoided in asthma.
- COPD patients are at greater risk of ischemic heart disease than asthmatics and they also have more severe airway obstruction. Cardioselective BBs are safe in patients with COPD who have an indication for their use.

- Calcium channel blockers—preferred choice for the treatment of hypertension in asthma
- Diuretics can be effectively used in OAD, but the potential for serious hypokalemia must be recognized with a concomitant inhaled beta-agonist.

MULTIPLE CHOICE QUESTIONS

1. Obstructive airway conditions include the following:
   A. Interstitial lung disease
   B. Pulmonary sarcoidosis
   C. Both
   D. None

2. Which of the following is a false statement?
   A. ACEI causes cough in patients with COPD
   B. ACEI causes cough in patients without any underlying respiratory condition
   C. ACEI causes frequent productive cough
   D. ACEI can aggravate bronchial asthma

3. In asthmatics, beta-blockers can cause the following:
   A. Increased bronchial obstruction
   B. Increased airway reactivity
   C. Resistance to effect of inhaled beta blocker receptor agonist
   D. All of the above

4. Preferred choice for treatment of hypertension in asthma:
   A. Diuretics
   B. Calcium channel blocker
   C. Beta-blockers
   D. ACEI

5. Side effects of amlodipine in elderly include:
   A. Fluid retention
   B. Constipation
   C. Both of them
   D. None of the above

Answers

1—D   2—C   3—D   4—B   5—C

REFERENCES

1. Morales DR, Jackson C, Lipworth BJ, Donnan PT, Guthrie B. Adverse respiratory effect of acute β-blocker exposure in asthma: a systematic review and meta-analysis of randomized controlled trials. Chest. 2014;145(4):779-86.
2. Salpeter S, Ormiston T, Salpeter E. Cardioselective beta-blocker use in patients with reversible airway disease. Cochrane Database Syst Rev. 2001;(2):CD002992.

SUGGESTED READINGS

1. Kaufman J, Schmitt S, Barnard J, Busse W. Angiotensin-converting enzyme inhibitors in patients with bronchial responsiveness and asthma. Chest. 1992;101(4):922-5.
2. Pinto B, Jadhav U, Singhai P, Sadhanandham S, Shah N. ACEI-induced cough: A review of current evidence and its practical implications for optimal CV risk reduction. Indian Heart J. 2020;72(5):345-50.
3. Morales DR, Lipworth BJ, Donnan PT, Wang H. Intolerance to angiotensin converting enzyme inhibitors in asthma and the general population: A UK Population-Based Cohort Study. J Allergy Clin Immunol Pract. 2021;9(9):3431-9.e4.

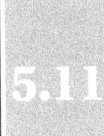

Resistant Hypertension

Amjad Khan

INTRODUCTION

Despite being one of the most prevalent conditions in the world, hypertension is still found to be poorly controlled and remains a common clinical problem faced by general physician as well as specialists. Uncontrolled blood pressure (BP) is positively associated with high risk for adverse cardiovascular events and is more likely to be due to secondary hypertension. The prevalence of resistant hypertension is higher in older patients as age and obesity are two important contributing factors.

DEFINITIONS

Resistant hypertension is defined as BP (readings based on accurate measurement techniques in accordance with current guidelines) that perpetually remains elevated above the target range for an individual in spite of simultaneous use of three or more than three antihypertensive agents of different drug classes commonly angiotensin-receptor blocker (ARB)/angiotensin-converting enzyme inhibitor (ACEI), long-acting calcium channel blocker (CCB) and thiazide/thiazide-like diuretic and shows poor response even with aggressive use of these drugs. Thus, by definition, patients who require four or more classes antihypertensive medicines including a diuretic for control of BP (<140/90 mm Hg) are known to have resistant hypertension. A diuretic should be added as one of the antihypertensive agents if its endured well by the patient and all of the prescribed drug agents should be given at maximum recommended (or maximally tolerated) antihypertensive dose at the appropriate time interval.

Apparent, True, and Pseudoresistant Hypertension

Resistant hypertension patients can further be classified into three types: True, pseudoresistant, and apparent hypertension.
1. *True resistant hypertension*: It is defined as having uncontrolled BP, confirmed by office BP >140/90 mm Hg based on average of at least two separate readings on two separate occasions and with a mean 24-hour ambulatory BP >130/80 mm Hg regardless of being compliant with an antihypertensive regimen that includes three or more drugs at their optimal doses which ideally includes at least one diuretic.

2. *Pseudoresistant hypertension*: Uncontrolled high BP that occurs not as a result of resistance to treatment but underlying factors that hinder or interfere with the treatment and cause false elevation in BP readings: The common causes of pseudoresistance are:
    - Inaccurate technique of BP measurement (e.g., inappropriately cuff size, an inadequately calibrated BP machine)
    - Poor adherence to antihypertensive therapy
    - Suboptimal antihypertensive therapy
    - Poor adherence to lifestyle and dietary approaches to lower BP, such as a reduced sodium intake
    - White-coat hypertension (WCH)
3. *Apparent resistant hypertension*: Apparent resistant hypertension in an individual is defined when pseudoresistant hypertension cannot be excluded or diagnosed either due to:
    - Lack of out office BP measurements such ambulatory blood pressure monitoring (ABPM) or home blood pressure monitoring (HBPM).
    - When important information regarding antihypertensive medication such as doses and adequacy of drug adherence is not available.
    - Uncertainty that three medicines were from three different antihypertensive drug class and one of them was a diuretic were taken by the patient at their maximally tolerated doses. Hence, in a patient with an office BP >140/90 mm Hg on ≥3 different classes antihypertensive medicines including a diuretic, who is not yet excluded of having pseudoresistant hypertension as a potential diagnosis, the term apparent resistant hypertension is preferred as some of these individuals might have true resistant, pseudoresistant, or secondary hypertension.
    - *WCH*: WCH is defined as office BP that averages to >140/90 mm Hg and reliable out-of-office 24-hour readings that is ABPM that averages <130/80 mm Hg or day time ABPM or HBPM that averages to <135/85 mm Hg, thus characterized by elevated clinic BP and normal out-of-office BP values. The main ethology behind WCH is anxiety and stress associated with visiting a doctor's office and having BP checked manually with a sphygmomanometer.

Refractory Hypertension

Refractory hypertension is defined as uncontrolled hypertension despite use of five or more drugs including chlorthalidone and a mineralocorticoid receptor antagonist under the care of a hypertension specialist.

In patients with resistant hypertension, isolated systolic hypertension is common along with frequent elevation in both SBP and DBP. In geriatric-resistant isolated systolic hypertension, treatment becomes difficult as increasing doses and frequency may lead to very low diastolic pressures.

EVALUATION

Assessment of medication adherence and optimal use of antihypertensive medication are the key in evaluation and diagnosis of patients with suspected resistant hypertension. Use of ABPM and HBPM is an essential step for accurate determination of BP needed to distinguish true and pseudoresistant hypertension as this distinction provides with an outline for further management which differs for different types of resistant hypertension. Identifying contributing factors for secondary hypertension and diagnosis of hypertension-mediated organ damage including retinopathy, left ventricular hypertrophy, and chronic kidney disease and assessment of comorbidities is important as it influences the antihypertensive treatment regimen.

MEDICAL HISTORY

The medical history should include the following: Onset, duration, progress, and severity of resistant hypertension. Details of present medications (naturopathy, alternative and over-the-counter medications) and side effects and allergic reaction to previous antihypertensive should be noted. True adherence to medicines can be established most accurately through questioning the patient. The physician should in a tactful manner ask about adverse effects caused after starting medication, number of missing doses in a week, and the reason for it such as financial and other socioeconomic stress, and other causes that may be responsible for limited adherence. History and clinical symptoms corresponding to secondary causes of hypertension, such as pheochromocytoma, Cushing syndrome, or obstructive sleep apnea should be inquired about.

PHYSICAL EXAMINATION

The physical examination should be directed towards the following: Adequate measurement of the BP according to the standard guidelines based on average of two BP readings taken at least after an interval of 5–10 minutes, diagnosis of secondary hypertension which is a potential cause of resistant hypertension, assessment of organ damage including funduscopic examination looking for retinopathy and pulse examination for peripheral vascular disease, auscultation of abdominal bruit examination for possible renovascular disease.

LABORATORY EVALUATION

The aim of laboratory evaluation is to rule out secondary causes of hypertension and hypertension-mediated organ damage and therefore following laboratory tests are recommended **(Box 1)**:
- Renal function test
- Serum electrolytes
- Blood sugar
- 24-hour urinalysis with estimation of proteinuria (e.g., urine albumin-to-creatinine ratio) should be obtained on patient's usual daily diet for sodium excretion analysis (provided not on diuretic in past 2 weeks), creatinine clearance, and aldosterone excretion.

Box 1: Basic testing in the patient with resistant hypertension.

- Ambulatory blood pressure monitoring
- 12-lead electrocardiogram
- Transthoracic echocardiogram
- Complete blood count
- Serum glucose, urea, creatinine, electrolytes, and lipids
- Urine analysis (protein, erythrocytes, leukocytes)
- 24-hour urine assessment for aldosterone, sodium, and albumin
- Plasma aldosterone concentration and renin
- Thyroid-stimulating hormone
- Renal echocardiogram
- Renal artery duplex

- Screening for primary aldosteronism is also recommended since, 11% fulfilled criteria for primary aldosteronism
  Paired morning measurement of the plasma aldosterone concentration (PAC) and plasma renin activity (PRA) is taken to look for elevated or high-normal PAC, suppressed PRA, and elevated PAC/PRA ratio. Certain antihypertensive drugs can alter the ratio. Hence, should be discontinued prior to testing.
- *Pheochromocytoma*: In presence of clinical symptoms including episodes of sudden spikes in BP, palpitations and/or diaphoresis, or tremor.

Noninvasive Imaging

Noninvasive imaging is particularly recommended for renal artery stenosis, important in patients with known atherosclerotic disease including peripheral artery disease, coronary artery disease, or cerebrovascular disease and patients with an abdominal bruit indicating obstructive renal artery disease.

A rise in serum creatinine after starting an ACE inhibitor or ARB. Young age onset of hypertension, which could be due to fibromuscular dysplasia. Because of low specificity, imaging studies are generally not recommended for screening of adrenal adenomas when biochemical tests are negative for hormonally active tumors.

TREATMENT

Nonpharmacologic Treatment

Nonpharmacologic treatment of resistant hypertension identification of factors contributing to resistant hypertension such as nonadherence to lifestyle interventions which involve dietary changes including low sodium diet and high fiber diet, at least 30 minutes of aerobic exercise, limiting alcohol consumption, and reducing weight to a healthy body mass index (BMI).

Patients diagnosed with secondary hypertension should be referred to appropriate specialist for treatment of the underlying cause, e.g., sleep specialist for management of obstructive sleep apnea which is usually managed by continuous positive airway pressure (CPAP). Medications that may be contributing to hypertension as a side effect should be withdrawn and avoided, if possible or at least the dosages should be reduced if the medication cannot be entirely stopped.

Pharmacological Treatment

By definition, the treatment for resistant hypertension includes at least three or more drugs, including a diuretic. The choice of agents should be customized and tailored to individual needs and demands and depends upon patient adherence, history of side effects and allergic reactions, financial limitations, and concomitant comorbidities including chronic kidney disease or diabetes or other metabolic disorders.

Regimens should be kept as simple as possible and long-acting combination agents are preferred to reduce the number of prescribed pills and avoid any confusion so that one single pill can be taken at a time. Treatment adherence worsens with increase in number of medicines, complexity of the dosing regimen, and financial strain. Medication-related adverse effects should be discussed, with down titration of or substitution for the offending agent.

- The pharmacologic treatment of resistant hypertension involves combinations of three or more drugs. Some patients have a specific indication for a class of drugs (e.g., beta blocker or nondihydropyridine CCB for rate control in atrial fibrillation). If there is no such indication, the preferred three-drug regimen consists of an ACE inhibitor or ARB, a long-acting CCB such as amlodipine, and a long-acting thiazide diuretic, preferably chlorthalidone. Among patients with an estimated glomerular filtration rate of <30 mL/min/1.73 m^2, a loop diuretic, such as furosemide or torsemide, is usually necessary for effective volume control.
- In patients with persistent uncontrolled hypertension despite the above three-drug regimen in optimal dose, spironolactone is typically began at 12.5 mg/day and titrate up to, but not above, 50 mg/day in the absence of proven primary aldosteronism. Monitoring of serum potassium levels for both hypokalemia and hyperkalemia are necessary if chlorthalidone and spironolactone are used. For patients who cannot tolerate spironolactone, eplerenone and amiloride are alternatives.
- In patients who are still hypertensive, vasodilating beta-blocker such as carvedilol can be considered. Alternatives include a long-acting, centrally acting agent such as guanfacine or a clonidine.
- Among patients who remain resistant, a direct vasodilator such as hydralazine for women or minoxidil for men may be used.

RENAL NERVE DENERVATION (FLOWCHART 1)

Preliminary data suggest that denervation of the renal sympathetic nerves (also known as renal nerve denervation), either by catheter-based

Confirm treatment resistance
- Office blood pressure >140/90 or 130/80 mm Hg in patients with diabetes or chronic kidney disease

and
- Patient prescribed three or more antihypertensive medications at optimal doss, including if possible a diuretic

or
- Office blood pressure at goal but patient requiring four or more antihypertensive medications

↓

Exclude pseudoresistance
- Is patient adherent with prescribed regimen?
- Obtain home, work, or ambulatory blood pressure readings to exclude white-coat effect

↓

Identify and reverse contributing lifestyle factors
- Obesity
- Physical inactivity
- Excessive alcohol ingestion
- High salt, low fiber diet

↓

Discontinue or minimize interfering substances
- Non-steroidal anti-inflammatory agents
- Sympathomimetics (diet pills, decongestant)
- Stimulants
- Oral contraceptives
- Licorice
- Ephedra

↓

Screen for secondary causes or hypertension
- Obstructive sleep apnea (snoring, witnessed apnea, excessive daytime sleepiness)
- Primary aldosteronism (elevated aldosterone one/renin ratio)
- Chronic kidney disease (creatinine clearance <30 mL/min)
- Renal artery stenosis (young female, known atherosclerotic disease, worsening real function)
- Pheochromocytoma (episodic hypertension, palpitations diaphoresis, headache)
- Cushing's syndrome (moon facies, central obesity, abdominal striae, inter-scapular fat deposition)
- Aortic coarctation (differential in brachial or femoral pulses, systolic bruit)

↓

Pharmacologic treatment
- Maximize diuretic therapy, including possible addition of mineralocorticoid receptor antagonist
- Combine agents with different mechanisms of action
- Use of loop diuretics in patients with chronic kidney disease and/or patients receiving potent vasodilator (e.g., minoxidil)

↓

Refer or specialist
- Refer to appropriate specialist for known or suspected secondary cause(s) of hypertension
- Refer to hypertension specialist if blood pressure remains uncontrolled after 6 months of treatment

FLOWCHART 1: Approach to resistant hypertension

radiofrequency ablation or by catheter-based ultrasound ablation, reduces BP in patients without resistant hypertension. In patients with resistant hypertension, the best data come from a large, blinded, randomized trial (SYMPLICITY-HTN-3) that failed to demonstrate benefit from renal nerve denervation compared with a sham procedure.

EXPERIMENTAL THERAPIES

Experimental therapies that have been evaluated include electrical stimulation of the carotid sinus baroreceptors and creation of a central arteriovenous anastomosis.

SUMMARY

Resistant hypertension is defined as BP that remains above target BP in spite of concurrent use of three antihypertensive agents of different classes and is more prevalent in elderly patients and secondary hypertension.

Resistant hypertension may be of true, pseudo, and apparent category. Pseudoresistant hypertension is due to suboptimal medications, lack of adherence to medications/lifestyle factors, and white-coat hypertension and inaccurate measurement of BP-resistant hypertension is evaluated by history, physical examination, laboratory investigation, and noninvasive imaging. It is managed conservatively by different classes of antihypertensive medication as well newer modalities such as renal artery denervation and central arteriovenous anastomosis.

MULTIPLE CHOICE QUESTIONS

1. Resistant hypertension is defined by failure of achievement of target BP by concurrent use of how many antihypertensive drug at optimum doses:
   A. 2
   B. 4
   C. 3
   D. 6

2. Pseudoresistant hypertension is commonly caused by:
   A. Inaccurate BP measurement
   B. Suboptimal antihypertensive therapy
   C. White-coat hypertension
   D. All of the above

3. Which of the following is a false statement?
   A. In white-coat hypertension, average office reading is >130/80 mm Hg
   B. In white-coat hypertension, average out-of-office reading is <130/80 mm Hg
   C. In white-coat hypertension, target organ damage is more severe
   D. All of the above

4. The preferred three-drug regimen consists of:
   A. ACEI, CCB, thiazide diuretic
   B. ACEI, CCB, loop diuretic
   C. ACEI, CCB, beta blocker
   D. ACEI, CCB, alpha blocker

5. Common investigation in resistant hypertension includes following, except:
   A. Renal artery duplex
   B. Renal angiography
   C. Renal echocardiogram
   D. Ambulatory BP monitoring

Answers

1—C 2—D 3—C 4—A 5—B

SUGGESTED READINGS

1. Azizi M, Sanghvi K, Saxena M, Gosse P, Reilly JP, Levy T, et al. Ultrasound renal denervation for hypertension resistant to a triple medication pill (RADIANCE-HTN TRIO): a randomised, multicentre, single-blind, sham-controlled trial. Lancet. 2021;397(10293):2476-86.
2. Bhatt DL, Kandzari DE, O'Neill WW, D'Agostino R, Flack JM, Katzen BT, et al. A controlled trial of renal denervation for resistant hypertension. N Engl J Med. 2014;370(15):1393-401.
3. Nuredini G, Saunders A, Rajkumar C, Okorie M. Current status of white coat hypertension: where are we? Ther Adv Cardiovasc Dis. 2020;14:1753944720931637.

CHAPTER 6

Overview of Guidelines on Management of Hypertension

Nihar Mehta, Zakiya E Patni

AIM

The primary aim of antihypertensive management is to effectively control blood pressure (BP) by reducing it to the target levels and to prevent, delay, and reverse progression of complications and risks associated with high BP, not only cardiovascular but the overall risk. Nonpharmacological approaches and lifestyle modifications are usually lifelong. Once drug therapy is initiated, compliance should be stressed upon. Antihypertensive management should be modified to an individual and his/her circumstances should be taken into consideration.

OBJECTIVES

According to the 2021 World Health Organization (WHO) hypertension guideline in adults.

The hypertension guideline objectives are as follows:
- To implement a threshold BP reading based on office, ambulatory, or home BP measurements for the initiation of hypertension treatment.
- To ascertain if laboratory investigations and/or cardiovascular risk assessment will be needed prior to initiation of pharmacological antihypertensive treatment.
- To decide the class of antihypertensive pharmacological agents with which to initiate therapy—and whether monotherapy, dual therapy, or single-pill combinations will be needed in a particular individual.
- To provide a target range of BP for hypertension control in an individual.
- To establish follow-up frequency and interval period after commencing treatment.
- To determine the role of nonphysician healthcare workers in the management and control of hypertension.

NONPHARMACOLOGICAL TREATMENT: LIFESTYLE MODIFICATIONS

Lifestyle modifications form the backbone of management of hypertension. In hypertensive individuals, they form the first line of treatment before initiating pharmacotherapy.

According to screening, diagnosis, assessment, and management of primary hypertension in adults in India, Ministry of Health and Family Welfare, Government of India.
- Grade I hypertension can be treated by making modification in lifestyle alone through dietary changes and aerobic exercise. Lifestyle interventions can also reduce overall cardiovascular mortality and morbidity and in patients who are on hypertensive, it aids to reduce down dosages.
- Patients with grade I hypertension on nonpharmacological therapy should be monitored for a duration of 1-3 months. In patients who are at high risk, lower range of duration should be considered before starting drug therapy. The interventions are summarized as follows.

Lifestyle Modifications (Table 1)

TABLE 1: Lifestyle modifications.

Salt reduction	• Reduce dietary sodium intake to <100 mmol/day <2.4 g sodium or <6 g salt (sodium chloride) • Reduce salt added when preparing foods and at the table. Avoid or limit consumption of high salt foods such as pickles, soy sauce, fast foods, and processed/packaged food including breads and cereals
Healthy diet	• Eating a diet that is rich in whole grains, fruits, vegetables, polyunsaturated fats, and dairy products and reducing food high in sugar, saturated fat, and trans fats • *DASH diet*: Eat diet rich in fruit, vegetables, low-fat dairy products. Eat less saturated and total fat • Other beneficial foods and nutrients include those high in magnesium, calcium, and potassium such as avocados, nuts, seeds, legumes, and tofu
Healthy drinks	• Moderate consumption of coffee, green and black tea • Other beverages that can be beneficial include arcadé (hibiscus) tea, pomegranate juice, beetroot juice, and cocoa
Moderation of alcohol consumption	• The recommended daily limit for alcohol consumptions is two standard drinks for men and 1.5 for women (10 g alcohol/standard drink) • Avoid binge drinking
Weight reduction	• Abdominal obesity should be managed • Ethnic-specific cut-offs for BMI and waist circumference should be used. (Ideal BMI 20–25 kg/m^2) • Alternatively, a waist-to-height ratio <0.5 is recommended for all populations
Smoking cessation	Total abstinence from smoking/tobacco in any form

Continued

Continued

Regular physical activity	• Moderate intensity aerobic exercise (walking, jogging, cycling, yoga, or swimming) for 30 minutes on 5–7 days/week • High-intensity interval training (HIIT) which involves alternating short bursts of intense activity with subsequent recovery periods of lighter activity • Strength training also can help reduce blood pressure. Performance of resistance/strength exercises on 2–3 days/week
Reduce stress and induce mindfulness	• Stress should be reduced and mindfulness or meditation introduced into the daily routine • Although more research is needed to determine the effects of chronic stress on blood pressure, randomized clinical trials suggest the beneficial effects of transcendental meditation/mindfulness on blood pressure
(BMI: body mass index, DASH: Dietary Approaches to Stop Hypertension)	

PHARMACOLOGICAL THERAPY

Blood Pressure Threshold for Initiation of Pharmacotherapy

Lifestyle modification advice should be given to all the patients.

- *High normal BP*: Initiate drug treatment of individuals without cardiovascular disease but with high cardiovascular risk, renal disease, and metabolic disorders, and systolic blood pressure (SBP) of 130–139 mm Hg (WHO guidelines, 2021)
- *Grade I hypertension*: Repeat readings should be taken at regular intervals in addition to nonpharmacological management. Pharmacotherapy is commenced after 3–6 months if the BP readings remain high in spite of lifestyle modification.

  Those patients who have evidence of existing cardiovascular disease, therapy should be started immediately.

  Pharmacotherapy should be initiated in individuals without any cardiovascular disease but with high risk of cardiovascular disease including coronary artery disease (CAD), heart failure, and valvular diseases. Therapy should also be commenced in diabetes mellitus (DM) or chronic kidney disease with three or more risk factors (such as age, gender, smoking, obesity, dyslipidemia, diabetes, impaired fasting glucose, and family history of heart issues).
- *Grade II or III hypertension*: Immediate drug therapy is recommended in addition to lifestyle modification.

Initiation of Blood Pressure-lowering Therapy as per Grade of Hypertension (ESC/ESH 2018) (Flowchart 1)

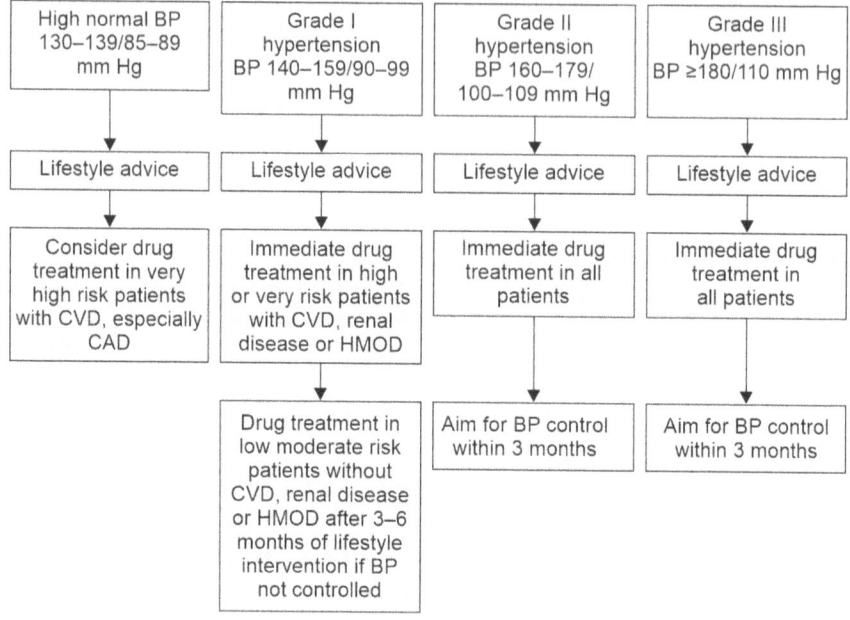

FLOWCHART 1: Initiation of BP lowering therapy.
(BP: blood pressure; CAD: coronary artery disease; CVD: cardiovascular disease; HMOD: hypertension-mediated organ damage)

Laboratory Testing Before Initiating Pharmacotherapy

Prior to commencing pharmacological therapy in hypertensive patients, it is highly recommended that certain tests and investigations be done keeping in mind that they do not delay treatment.

Routine Investigations

Routine laboratory tests are recommended before initiating therapy for high BP to:
- *Guide treatment*: To help chose one medication over the other
- To diagnose secondary hypertension
- To diagnose presence of other comorbidities, e.g., DM and dyslipidemia
- To determine end organ or tissue damage, e.g., chronic kidney disease (CKD) and left ventricular hypertrophy (LVH)
- To evaluate cardiovascular risk factors. These laboratory tests include:
  ○ Hemoglobin and hematocrit
  ○ Blood urea nitrogen (BUN), creatinine, and estimated glomerular filtration rate (eGFR)
  ○ Serum sodium and potassium
  ○ Fasting lipid profile

CHAPTER 6 Overview of Guidelines on Management of Hypertension

- Fasting blood sugar (FBS), postprandial blood sugar (PPBS), and glycosylated hemoglobin (HbA1c)
- Urine routine/microscopy. Urine dipstick test for proteins
- Electrocardiogram (ECG)

Additional testing in an individual is based upon presence of clinical features, presence of modifiable and unmodifiable risk factors, diagnosis of comorbidities, and diagnosis of hypertension-mediated organ damage (HMOD).

Pharmacotherapy: Determining Initial Antihypertensive Therapy (Flowchart 2)

- Drug classes recommended as first-line treatment for stage I/II hypertension include:
  - ACE inhibitors
  - Angiotensin-receptor blockers
  - Calcium channel blockers
  - Diuretics
- Additional classes of drugs include:
  - Mineralocorticoid receptor antagonists
  - Newer β-blockers
  - Alpha blockers
  - Centrally acting agents

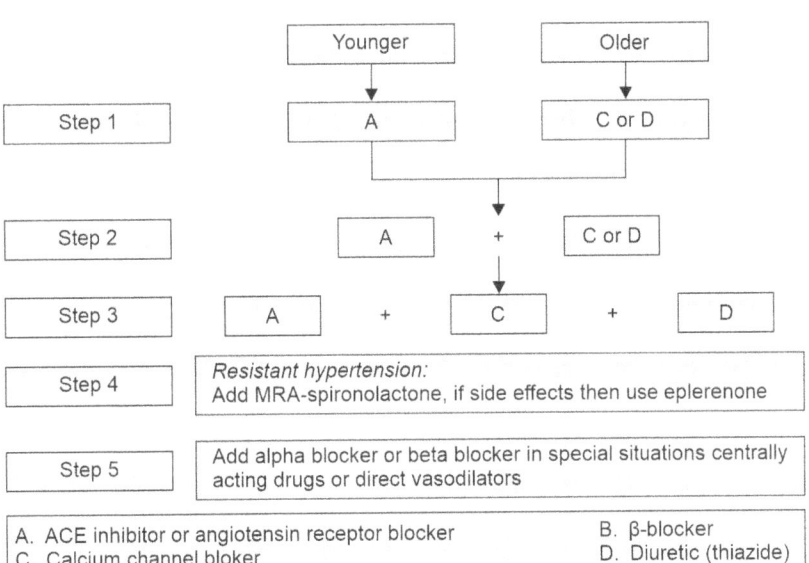

FLOWCHART 2: Algorithm for pharmacotherapy for hypertension.
(MRA: mineralocorticoid receptor antagonist)

- An antihypertensive agent should be determined keeping in mind the age of the patient, associated modifiable and nonmodifiable risk factors, presence of HMOD, comorbidities, social and economic conditions, accessibility of the drug, and finally the better judgement of the physician based on their experience.
- The type of antihypertensive therapy is determined by patient's BP and how far is it above target level. If the BP reading is >20 mm Hg systolic and 10 mm Hg diastolic blood pressure (DBP) above target range for a specific individual, the standard antihypertensive management is that they are to be started on a two-drug therapy, either as a single pill combination or two different pills.
- *Combination therapy*: Antihypertensive drugs when used in combination of two or more drugs in low dosages produce synergistic effect and are known to show lesser side effects.
- In about 70% of hypertensive patients on pharmacotherapy, the BP targets are achieved with dual therapy or addition of more only WHO recommends combination therapy, initially as a single-pill combination in adults with high BP. It is especially indicated when the baseline BP is ≥20 mm Hg systolic/10 mm Hg diastolic higher than the target BP and is considered more valuable and effective in such patients.
- When determining the class of antihypertensive drugs with which to initiate treatment, the foremost commonly used drugs which are considered are ACEI/ARB, long-acting CCBs, and diuretics (thiazide or thiazide-like).
- Use of fixed dose formulations/single-pill combinations is encouraged to improve compliance.
- Use of long-acting drugs that provide 24-hour efficacy helps to improve patient compliance as they require only one time administration.
- Although antihypertensive therapy once initiated has to be taken lifelong, an effort can be made to decrease the dosage and number of medicines once BP target levels are achieved and the patient is clear of any potential threat in term of organ damage, sudden BP fluctuations leading to hypertensive emergency (step-down therapy).
- Alteration in drug dosages may be needed based on seasonal variation as BP tends to be lower at higher temperatures and higher at lower temperatures.

Indications and Contraindications of First Line Antihypertensive Drugs (Table 2)

TABLE 2: Indications and contra-indications of first line antihypertensive drugs.

Class of drugs	Definite indication/s	Possible indication/s	Definite contraindication/s	Relative contraindication/s
Diuretics	• Heart failure • Elderly patients • Systolic hypertension	Diabetes	Gout	Dyslipidemia

Continued

Continued

Class of drugs	Definite indication/s	Possible indication/s	Definite contraindication/s	Relative contraindication/s
CCBs	• Metabolic syndrome • Angina • Elderly • Systolic hypertension • Diabetes	Peripheral vascular disease CVA	Heart block[a]	Congestive heart failure[a]
ACEIs	• Metabolic syndrome • Heart failure • Left ventricular dysfunction • Postmyocardial infarction • Significant proteinuria • Diabetes	CVA	• Pregnancy and lactation • Bilateral renal artery stenosis • Hyperkalemia	Moderate renal failure (creatinine levels >3 mg/dL)
ARBs	• Metabolic syndrome • Diabetes mellitus • Proteinuria • LV dysfunction • ACEI-induced cough	Heart failure CVA	• Pregnancy and lactation • Bilateral renal artery stenosis • Hyperkalemia	Moderate renal failure (creatinine levels >3 mg/dL)

[a]Verapamil or diltiazem
(ACEI: angiotensin-converting enzyme inhibitor; ARB: angiotensin receptor blocker; CCB: calcium channel blocker; CVA: cerebrovascular accident; LV: left ventricular)

Indications and Contraindications of Other Antihypertensive Drugs (Table 3)

TABLE 3: Indications and contraindications of other antihypertensive drugs

Class of drugs	Definite Indication/s	Possible indication/s	Definite contraindication/s	Relative contraindication/s
β-blockers	• Angina • Postmyocardial infarction • Tachyarrhythmia • Heart failure	• Pregnancy • Diabetes	Heart block	• Dyslipidemia • Physically active • Peripheral vascular disease • Elderly persons >50 years • Asthma and chronic pulmonary disease (COPD)

Continued

Continued

Class of drugs	Definite Indication/s	Possible indication/s	Definite contra-indication/s	Relative contraindication/s
α blockers (doxazosin and prazosin)	• Prostatic hypertrophy • Chronic kidney disease (CKD)	• Glucose intolerance • Dyslipidemia	• Orthostatic hypotension • Congestive heart failure	
Centrally acting agents:				
α methyl-dopa	Hypertension in pregnancy	Resistant hypertension	Acute or chronic liver disease	
Clonidine	Resistant hypertension	CKD	Pregnancy and lactation	
Vasodilators (hydralazine)	• Resistant hypertension • Hypertension in pregnancy			Coronary artery disease

Adverse Effects of Major Classes of Antihypertensive Drugs (Table 4)

TABLE 4: Adverse effects of major classes of antihypertensive drugs.

Common side effects	ACEI	ARB	Calcium channel blocker	Diuretic	β-blocker
Headache	–	–	+	–	–
Flushing	–	–	+	–	–
Lethargy	–	–	–	–	+
Impotence	–	–	–	+	+
Dry cough	+	+/–	–	–	–
Gout	–	–	–	+	–
Edema	–	–	+	–	–
Postural hypotension	+	+	–	+	–
Cold hands and feet	–	–	–	–	+
Hyperkalemia	+	+	–	–	–
Hyperglycemia				+	+
Dyslipidemia				+	+
Angioedema	+	+			

(ACEI: angiotensin-converting enzyme inhibitor; ARB: angiotensin receptor blocker)

Target of Therapy

- BP control should be individualized based on the age, activity, risk factors, and concomitant diseases.
- The first objective of treatment should be to reduce the BP to <140/90 mm Hg in all patients. If the treatment is well-tolerated, the BP should be brought down to 130/80 mm Hg in most patients.
- DBP should be targeted at below 80 mm Hg in all patients, irrespective of age and risk factors.
- *Age <65 years*: The target BP should be 120-130 mm Hg, especially in patients at high cardiovascular risk.
- *Age >65 years*: The target BP should be 130-140 mm Hg.
- *Patients with established CAD or heart failure*: The target BP should be 120-130 mm Hg.
- In frail elderly patients, especially those who are inactive or have postural hypotension, high BP targets should be accepted.
- BP control should not be <120/70 mm Hg since below this level, the risk may be higher.
- It should be recognized that BP has wide variations and most BP readings should be within the range prescribed, fully understanding that some reading could fluctuate in either direction.
- SBP continues to rise throughout life. Conversely, DBP rises until approximately 50 years of age following which it remains the same or falls with age. Diastolic hypertension predominates before the age of 50 years (isolated or along with systolic hypertension).
- DBP is a more potent risk factor until age the 50 years. SBP, at any age, is a major cardiovascular risk factor and warrants greater attention.
- BP thresholds to start treatment and target BP to be achieved [Indian Guidelines on Hypertension-IV (IGH IV) 2019] **(Table 5)**.

TABLE 5: Threshold to start treatment and target BP range.

Subjects	Threshold to start treatment (≥)	Target BP range
Age <65 years		
High ASCVD risk	140/90	120–130/70–80
Low ASCVD risk	140/90	130–140/70–80
Age 65–80 years	140/90	130–140/70–80
Age >80 years	140–150/90	130–140/70–80
With other risk factors		
Diabetes	140/90	130–140/70–80
History of stroke, TIA	140/90	130–140/70–80
Chronic kidney disease	140/90	130–140/70–80
Coronary artery disease	130/80	120–130/70–80
Heart failure	130/80	120–130/70–80

(ASCVD: atherosclerotic cardiovascular disease; BP: blood pressure; TIA: transient ischemic attack)

Follow-up Frequency and Interval

The patient is advised follow-up based on BP reading and response to antihypertensive therapy and how rigorously lifestyle interventions are followed.
- If target BP achieved:
  - Follow-up in every 3 months (high risk and very high risk)
  - Follow-up in every 6 months (medium and low risk)
- If target BP is not achieved within 1 month:
  - In case of partial response, consider adding a drug from another class with increase in the dose of the current antihypertensive.
  - In case target BP is still not achieved, consider use of three pharmacological agents. Single-pill combination of three antihypertensive drugs can be used if it is easily available.
- In occurrence of side effects:
  - Consider substitution with a drug from a different drug class or low-dose combination from another class.
  - Reduce dose of the current ongoing drug with addition of a drug from another class.
- If hypertension is becomes difficult to manage, refer to a specialist.

ASSOCIATED THERAPIES

Hypertensive patients often have several other associated comorbidities that increase the cardiovascular risk.
- *Aspirin*: As additional therapy does not have an effect on high BP unless atherosclerotic cardiovascular disease (ASCVD) is present. Studies based on prevention trials known as ASCEND, ARRIVE, and the ASPREE trial were conducted to understand the role of aspirin for primary prevention in elderly (ARRIVE and ASPREE) and diabetic (ASCEND) individuals. These studies concluded that aspirin did not show benefit in prevention and management of hypertension unless associated with atherosclerosis.
- As a secondary prevention in hypertensive patients with CAD or ASCVD risk, aspirin can be prescribed. Statins are prescribed as a secondary prevention in all hypertensive patients with coronary, peripheral, or cerebrovascular disease with dyslipidemia having low-density lipoprotein (LDL) levels >100 mg/dL.
- Among statins rosuvastatin given in a dose of 10 mg/day has proven to be more beneficial than antihypertensive drugs in hypertensive patients with high risk of cardiovascular conditions. Evidence shows that even in the absence of cardiovascular diseases, as a primary prevention in high risk patients, statins should be started based on the recent study published, HOPE III, trial in hypertensive patients.

NEWER MODALITIES

- Carotid baroreceptor stimulation therapy has been studied more in depth in recent years. The mechanism involves stimulating baroreceptors

through an implanted device. The principal group for which the therapy is indicated is resistant hypertension patients as it has shown significant reduction in BP. The therapy is in its experimental stages and clinical application has not been approved yet.
- *Renal sympathetic denervation therapy*: The mechanism involves radiofrequency ablation of sympathetic plexus around the renal arteries by using special catheters. However, renal denervation therapy is still under evaluation as SIMPLICITY III trial which was conducted recently did not show any significant effect on BP reduction and therefore remains inapplicable for BP management.
- Creation of an arteriovenous (AV) anastomosis between the external iliac artery and vein using a fixed caliber stent such as nitinol device (ROX arteriovenous coupler) diverts blood from the arterial to the venous system and results in an immediate reduction of BP. This is still not approved for routine clinical use.

Comparisons of Various Guidelines (Table 6)

TABLE 6: Comparisons of Various Guidelines

Guidelines	ESC/ESH 2018	ISH 2020	IGH IV 2019
Target for starting treatment	• In high risk for CV disease 130–139/85–89 • In grade I hypertension with low risk for HMOD treatment to be commenced after lifestyle intervention fails	• If BP >140–150/90–99 mm Hg • Start lifestyle intervention followed by drugs • In grade II hypertension >160/100 start drugs immediately with lifestyle modification	• Threshold is 140/90 for most patients • In CAD 130/80 • HF <130/80 • *In stage 1 hypertension*: Repeat readings within 2–3 weeks with lifestyle modification and pharmacotherapy to be started withIn 1 month • *In stage 2/3*: Shorter waiting period for pharmacotherapy • In HMOD/ASCVD pharmacotherapy to be started earliest
Treatment	Recommended two-drugs combination in SPC	• Use any drugs available and include as many of those below as possible • Consider monotherapy in grade I and age >80 years or frail	Younger: • *Step 1*: ACEI/ARB • *Step 2*: ACEI/ARB + CCB/diuretics • *Step 3*: ACEI/ARB + CCB + Diuretics • *Step 4*: Resistant hypertension

Continued

Continued

Guidelines	ESC/ESH 2018	ISH 2020	IGH IV 2019
	If resistant hypertension: add spironolactone, or if resistant to it add eplerenone, amiloride, thiazide-like, loop diuretic or add bisoprolol/doxazosin	Simplify dosing with once-daily dosing and SPC *Non-black patients*: Low dose ARB/ACE +DHP-CCB Increase dose/add thiazide-like diuretics/spironolactone/amiloride/eplerenone/clonidine/beta-blocker *Black patients*: Low dose ARB + DHP-CCB or DHP-CCB + thiazide/thiazide-like increase to full dose Or add ARB/ACE Or add spironolactone/amiloride /doxazosin/eplerenone/clonidine/beta-blocker	*Add MRA*: Spironolactone if nontolerated, use eplerenone *Step 5*: Add alpha-blocker or beta-blocker in special situations Centrally acting drugs or direct vasodilators Older Step 1 CCB/diuretics Rest steps same.
(ACEI: angiotensin-converting enzyme inhibitor; ARB: angiotensin receptor blocker; ASCVD: atherosclerotic cardiovascular disease; CAD: coronary artery disease; CCB: calcium channel blocker; DHP: dihydropyridine; ESC: European Society of Cardiology; ESH: European Society of Hypertension; HF: heart failure; HMOD: hypertension-mediated organ damage; ISH: International Society of Hypertension; IGH IV: Indian Guidelines on Hypertension-IV; MRA: magnetic resonance angiography; SPC: single-pill combination)			

Recommendation on Treatment by Nonphysician Professionals

According to WHO guidelines, pharmacological antihypertensive treatment by nonphysician healthcare professional depends upon local regulations which vary by country as long as the following conditions are met:
- Proper training
- Prescribing authority
- Specific management protocols
- Physician oversight

Community healthcare workers (HCWs) may assist in tasks such as:
- *Education*: Hypertension-related patient education is a part of antihypertensive management and should be stressed upon time and again. This can be accomplished by nonphysician professionals through aids such as leaflets and counseling.
- *Delivery of medications*: Antihypertensive medications are typically taken lifelong and regular BP check-up is important to determine their effectiveness. Checking BP without regular medication is impractical.

Nonphysician professional can help ensure the need for regular administration of antihypertensive drug therapy.
- *BP measurement and monitoring*: Measurement of BP with a mercury sphygmomanometer is considered a gold standard. Digital BP devices are now widely used in clinic settings as well as in home settings. Nonphysician staff can help ensure BP measurements are taken accurately by preventing any conditions that may result in fallacies in BP measurement and consequently result in discrepancies in BP readings.

SUMMARY

- The aim of antihypertensive management is to effectively reduce BP to target level and diagnose complications at the earliest for better and desired prognosis.
- *Nonpharmacological therapy*: Lifestyle interventions assist not only to lower down BP readings consequently reducing drug dosages but also bring down the overall cardiovascular risk.
- *Pharmacotherapy for hypertension*: Grade I hypertension (office BP ≥140-159/90-99 mm Hg), even without suspected HMOD, should now receive drug treatment if their BP is not within target range after 3-6 months of lifestyle intervention. For high-risk patients, with grade I hypertension and grades II and III hypertension (office BP ≥160/100 mm Hg), it is recommended that drug treatment be initiated immediately alongside lifestyle interventions.
- *Target of BP*: This has been a frequently debated topic. Evidence shows that lowering office SBP to <140 mm Hg is beneficial for all patient groups, including independent older patients. There is also evidence to support targeting SBP to 130 mm Hg for most patients, if tolerated. Even lower SBP levels (<130 mm Hg) will be tolerated and potentially beneficial for patients with CAD or heart failure. SBP should not be targeted to <120 mm Hg because the balance of benefit versus harm becomes concerning at these levels of treated SBP. Optimal DBP is <80 mm Hg. Treatment of elevated SBP should be continued even with low DBP.
- BP targets especially in old (≥65 years) is 130-139 mm Hg. In frail elderly patients, especially those who are inactive or have postural hypotension, high BP targets should be accepted.
- Combination therapy has the advantage of producing lesser side effects as low doses of two or more drugs having synergistic effect. In 70% of patients, goal blood pressure will be achieved with two or more agents only.
- Use of fixed-dose formulations/single-pill combinations is encouraged to improve compliance.
- A simplified drug treatment algorithm can be followed for drug therapy. An ACEI or ARB with a CCB or thiazide/thiazide-like diuretic is the usual combination therapy recommended for most patients. For those requiring three drugs, the recommended combination is pairing an ACEI or ARB with a CCB and a thiazide/thiazide-like diuretic. Spironolactone is the mineralocorticoid receptor antagonist of choice that should be added

in when needed depending upon the specific condition (e.g., angina, postmyocardial infarction, heart failure with reduced ejection fraction (HFrEF), tachycardia, or irregular heart rate).
- Aspirin is not required in hypertension unless associated with cardiovascular disease and stroke as a secondary prevention.
- Device-based therapy for the treatment of hypertension due to lack of information and evidence of safety and efficacy of device-based therapy; they are not recommended as of now.
- Newer therapies should be taken into consideration in cases of resistant BP. These include carotid baroreceptor stimulation therapy, renal sympathetic denervation therapy, and creating AV anastomosis.

MULTIPLE CHOICE QUESTIONS

1. Which antihypertensive drug class is contraindicated in hyperkalemia?
   A. CCB
   B. ACEI/ ARB
   C. Diuretic
   D. All of the above

2. Preferred statin of choice as secondary prevention in hypertensive patients?
   A. Atorvastatin
   B. Rosuvastatin
   C. Pravastatin
   D. Lovastatin

3. In a patient with gout and dyslipidemia following antihypertensive drug class is contraindicated.
   A. ACEI
   B. ARB
   C. Diuretic
   D. All of the above

4. Which of the following centrally acting agent can be used in pregnancy?
   A. α-Methyldopa
   B. Clonidine
   C. Both
   D. None

5. Which of the following is a false statement
   A. Initiate immediate antihypertensive drug therapy in grade II BP
   B. Initiate immediate antihypertensive drug therapy in patients with high CVD risk in grade I BP
   C. Initiate immediate antihypertensive drug therapy in high normal BP without CVD risk
   D. None

Answers

1—B 2—B 3—C 4—A 5—C

SUGGESTED READINGS

1. Ministry of Health and Family Welfare Government of India. (2016). Standard Treatment Guidelines. Hypertension Screening, Diagnosis, Assessment, and Management of Primary Hypertension in Adults in India. [online] Available from: http://clinicalestablishments.gov.in/WriteReadData/6591.pdf. [Last accessed December, 2022].
2. Flack JM, Adekola B. Blood pressure and the new ACC/AHA hypertension guidelines. Trends Cardiovasc Med. 2020;30(3):160-4.
3. Shah SN, Munjal YP, Kamath SA, Wander GS, Mehta N, Mukherjee S, et al. Indian Guidelines on Management of Hypertension (I.G.H) – IV 2019. J Hum Hypertens. 2020;34(11):745-58.
4. Munjal YP, Maiya M, Wander GS, Mehta N. Indian Guidelines on Management of Hypertension (I.G.H) – IV 2019. J Assoc Physicians India. 2019;67(9):1-48.
5. Williams B, Mancia G, Spiering W, Agabiti Rosei E, Azizi M, Burnier M, et al. 2018 ESC/ESH Guidelines for the management of arterial hypertension. The Task Force for the management of arterial hypertension of the European Society of Cardiology (ESC) and the European Society of Hypertension (ESH). Eur Heart J, 2018;39(33):3021-104.
6. Unger T, Borghi C, Charchar F, Khan NA, Poulter NR, Prabhakaran D, et al. 2020 International Society of Hypertension Global Hypertension Practice Guidelines. Hypertension. 2020;75(6):1334-57.
7. Whelton PK, Carey RM, Aronow WS, Casey Jr DE, Collins KJ, Himmelfarb CD, et al. 2017 ACC/AHA/AAPA/ABC/ACPM/AGS/APhA/vASH/ASPC/NMA/PCNA Guideline for the prevention, detection, evaluation, and management of high blood pressure in adults. Hypertension. 2018;71(6):e13-115.
8. World Health Organization. Guideline for the pharmacological treatment of hypertension in adults. Geneva: World Health Organisation; 2021. License: CC BY-NC-SA 3.0 IGO.

Index

Page numbers followed by *b* refer to box, *f* refer to figure, and *t* refer to table

A

Accelerated hypertension, treatment of 90, 90t
Accurate blood pressure
    check-up 8
    measurement 5
Acebutolol 48
Acetazolamide 45
Acromegaly 3
Acute coronary syndrome 77, 112
Adenosine triphosphatase 57
Adho mukha vrksasana 27
Adrenal 32
    steroids 3
    tumors 20
Adrenergic crisis 78
Advanced glycation end products 81
Alcohol 26
    consumption, moderation of 130
Aldosterone 32, 32t
Aldosteronism, primary 3, 21
Aliskiren 35
Alpha-blockers 53-55, 133, 136
Alpha-methyldopa 53, 55, 136
Ambulatory blood pressure
    measurement 10, 10f, 11t
    monitoring 2, 122
American College of Cardiology 1, 109
American Diabetes Association 80
American Heart Association 1, 109
Amiloride 43, 44
Amlodipine 38-40, 75
Angina 135
Angioedema 33, 136
Angiotensin–converting enzyme
    inhibitors 31-33, 39, 44, 67, 77, 82, 85, 90, 92, 102, 112, 113, 116, 118, 121, 133, 135, 136, 140
        contraindications of 34, 34b
        pharmacologic characteristics of 33, 33t
        side effects of 33, 33b
Angiotensin-receptor blockers 31, 34, 34t, 39, 44, 82, 90, 96, 102, 112, 113, 116, 118, 121, 133, 135, 136, 140
Ankle brachial index 5, 21, 110
Antagonists 45
Antihypertensive 53, 118
    classes of 53t
    drugs 89t, 134, 134t, 135, 135t
        major classes of 136, 136t
    therapy 71, 133
Antinatriuresis 32
Aorta
    coarctation of 20, 21
    evaluation of 21
Aortic aneurysm, abdominal 1
Aortic dissection 4, 77
Aortic stenosis, severe 34
Apoptosis 32
Appetite suppressants 3
Aquaretics 43-45
Arginine vasopressin receptor 43, 45
Arrhythmias 4, 20, 43
Arterial baroreceptors 60
Arterial vasodilator 105
Arteriovenous fistula 61
Artery, peripheral 19
Aspirin 138, 142
Asthma 116, 135
    chronic obstructive pulmonary disease overlap syndrome 118
    mild 50
    severe 50
Asymptomatic hypertension-mediated target organ damage 111
Atenolol 48, 90
Atherogenesis 32
Atheroma formation 32

Atherosclerosis 32
Atherosclerotic cardiovascular disease 137, 138, 140
Atherosclerotic renal occlusion 20
Atrial fibrillation 4, 19-21
Automated sphygmomanometer 6, 7f
Averapamil 135
Azilsartan 34
Azotemia 43
Back pain 59

B

Baroreceptor activation therapy 57
Benidipine 39
Beta-blockers 48-50, 77, 112, 117
　　effects of 48
　　pharmacologic properties of 48, 48t
Bisoprolol 49
Blood pressure 1, 9f, 11t, 20, 24, 31, 32, 40, 57, 60, 65, 70, 71, 77, 81, 82, 88, 90, 94, 104, 111, 121, 129, 131, 132, 137
　　control of 112
　　diastolic 1, 2, 60, 70, 81, 82, 109, 113
　　high 1, 2t, 65, 131
　　low 31
　　lowering therapy, initiation of 132
　　management, perioperative 103
　　measurement 5, 9, 9t, 10, 141
　　monitoring 141
　　normal 1, 131
　　out-of-office measurement of 10
　　patterns of 11t
　　systolic 1, 2, 58, 60, 70, 81, 82, 109, 113
　　target of 141
Blood sugar 123
　　fasting 21, 133
Blood urea nitrogen 21, 132
Blurred vision scotoma 89
Body mass index 20, 25, 124, 131
Bradycardia 50
　　severe 50
Bradykinin 32, 33
　　degradation 32
Brain 19
Breathlessness 19
Bronchospasm 50
Bumetanide 43, 44

C

Café-au-lait patches 20
Calcium channel blocker 38, 38t, 77, 82, 85, 89, 104, 117, 133, 135, 140
　　long-acting 121
　　pharmacological properties of 39, 39t
Candesartan 34
Captopril 33, 75
Carbonic anhydrase inhibitors 45
Cardiac arrest, sudden 32
Cardiac fibrosis 32
Cardiomyopathy, hypertrophic obstructive 34
Cardiovascular disease 1, 4, 65, 80, 110, 132
Carotid
　　baroreceptor
　　　　activation therapy 60
　　　　stimulation therapy 138
　　femoral pulse wave velocity 5
　　intima-media thickness 5
　　plaques 4
　　revascularization 19
　　ultrasound 5
Carteolol 48
Carvedilol 49
Central aortic blood pressure 14
Central nervous system 50, 74, 89
Cerebral hemorrhage 89
Cerebrovascular accident 21, 80, 135
Cerebrovascular disease 4, 5, 70
Chest
　　pain 19
　　X-ray of 75
Chloride 43
Chlorthalidone 43, 44
Chronic obstructive pulmonary disease 116, 118
Cilnidipine 39
Claudication 19
　　worsening of 50
Clonidine 53, 75, 89, 136
Cocaine 3
Coffee contains caffeine 26
Cold
　　extremities 50
　　feet 136
　　hands 136

Community healthcare workers 140
Complete blood count 75
Computed tomography 5, 21, 22
    scan 94
Conivaptan 43
Continuous positive airway pressure 125
Contraction, stimulation of 32
Convulsion 88
Coronary artery disease 19, 32, 112, 116, 131, 132, 137, 140
Cortical blindness 89
C-reactive protein 66
Creatinine 132
Cuff sizes 6*t*
Cushing syndrome 3, 21
    features of 20
Cyclosporine 3
Cysts, renal 3
Cytochrome P 39

D

Death 80
Deep tendon reflex 91
Dementia 19
Depression 50
    severe 50
Diabetes mellitus 12, 36, 50, 65, 80, 110, 131, 134, 135
    acute complications of 80
    type 1 81
    type 2 65
Diabetic ketoacidosis 80
Dietary sodium 25
Dihydropyridine 38*t*, 39, 140
Diltiazem 38, 39, 135
Dimethylarginine
    asymmetrical 96
    dimethylamine hydrolase 96
Distal convoluted tubule 42, 43
Diuretics 42, 118, 133
    classes of 43, 43*t*
    pharmacological characteristics of 44, 44*t*
Dizziness 43
Doxazosin 53, 136
Drug therapy 29
Dry cough 33, 136

Dual renin–angiotensin–aldosterone system 112
Dysautonomia, familial 3
Dyslipidemia 50, 65, 111, 132, 134-136

E

Echocardiogram 111
Eclampsia 88
    treatment of 91
Edema 136
    acute pulmonary 77
    feet 19
    peripheral 84
    pulmonary 88
Efonidipine 39
Electrocardiogram 5, 75, 111, 133
Elevated jugular venous pressure 84
Enalapril 33, 76
Enalaprilat 33, 104
Endothelial dysfunction 32
Endothelin 96
Endothelium 32
Eplerenone 43, 44, 86
Eprosartan 34
Erectile dysfunction 19, 50
Erythropoietin 3
Esmolol 49, 76, 104
Estimated glomerular filtration rate 5, 21, 82, 98, 110, 111, 132
Estrogens, high-dose 3
European Society of Cardiology 1, 61, 109, 140
European Society of Hypertension 1, 140
Extracellular fluid 96
Eye 4, 19

F

Fatigue 50
Felodipine 39
Femoral artery pseudoaneurysm 59
Fenoldopam 104
Fibrinogen 32
Fibromuscular dysplasia 3, 20, 22
Fibrosis 32
Fimasartan 34

Frequent nocturnal hemodialysis 98
Fundoscopy 5, 20, 21
Furosemide 43, 44

G

Gangrene 19, 50
Glomerular fibrosis 32
Glomerular filtration rate 89, 95, 95f, 97
Glucocorticoid remediable hypertension 3
Glucose 136
    intolerance 32
    transport 66
Gordon syndrome 3
Gout 131, 134, 136
Guanabenz 53
Guanfacine 53
Guideline-directed medical therapy 86

H

Head, computed tomography of 75
Headache 19, 89, 136
Heart 19, 20, 32
    block 50, 135
    disease, ischemic 77, 109, 112, 112t
    failure 1, 19, 43, 50, 54, 84, 85, 105, 131, 134, 135, 137, 140
        acute 85
        chronic 85
        congestive 77, 136
        with left ventricular ejection fraction 84
        with preserved ejection fraction 4
        with reduced ejection fraction 84, 142
        worsening of 50
    rate, irregular 142
    sound 20
Hematocrit 132
Hemoglobin 132
    glycosylated 21, 80, 133
Hemolysis, elevated liver enzymes, low platelet count 89

Hemorrhage
    intracranial 70
    subarachnoid 71
Henle loop 42
Hepatic dysfunction 89
High-density lipoprotein 50
    cholesterol 65
Home blood pressure
    measurement 10
    monitoring 2, 13, 122
Hormone, antidiuretic 42
Hydralazine 53, 55, 76, 89, 91, 104, 136
Hydrochlorothiazide 43, 44
Hydroxyindoleacetic acid 75
Hydroxylase deficiency 3
Hydroxysteroid dehydrogenase deficiency 3
Hypercalcemia 3
Hyperglycemia 43, 136
Hyperinsulinemia 66
Hyperkalemia 33, 34, 135, 136
Hyperosmolar hyperglycemic state 80
Hypersensitivity 34
Hypertension 2, 10, 12f, 12t, 18-21, 24, 25, 39, 43, 45, 65, 67, 70, 80, 84, 85, 88, 90, 91, 94, 97, 109, 116, 129, 131, 133, 136
    association of 85
    chronic 88
    complications of 88, 88t
    control 98
    essential 20, 20t
    gestational 88
    management of 85, 97, 112, 116, 129
    mediated organ damage 4, 18-21, 132, 133, 140
        evaluation of 4t
    pathogenesis of 94
    pathophysiology of 81
    perioperative 101
    pharmacotherapy for 133, 141
    pregnancy-induced 77
    prevalence of 116
    primary 2
    pseudoresistant 121, 122
    refractory 122

resistant 60, 121, 122, 124b, 126b, 127, 136
risks of 4
screening for 14
secondary 2, 3, 20, 21, 21t
severe 74, 78
systemic 57, 109-111, 112t
systolic 134, 135
treatment of 81
true resistant 121
Hypertensive crisis 43
Hypertensive emergency 74, 75, 78
drugs for 76t
Hyperthyroidism 3, 20
Hyperuricemia 43
Hyponatremia 33
Hypotension 34
orthostatic 33, 136
postural 136
Hypothalamus, paraventricular nucleus of 58
Hypothyroidism 3, 20
Hypovolemia 43

I

Impaired fasting glucose 82
Impaired glucose tolerance 82
Impotence 43, 136
Indapamide 43, 44
Indian Guidelines on Hypertension 1, 140
Insomnia 50
International Society of Hypertension 140
Interstitial fibrosis 32
Intracranial pressure 3, 77
Intraglomerular pressure 32
Irbesartan 34
Ischemic heart disease 77, 109, 112, 112t
prevalence of 109, 109t, 111

K

Kidney 19, 21, 32
disease 4, 5
chronic 4, 5, 12, 25, 36, 80, 94, 95, 95f, 97, 98, 132, 136, 137
palpable 20
sympathetic reinnervation of 59
K-sparing diuretics 43, 44

L

Labetalol 49, 71, 75-78, 90, 103, 105
Lacidipine 40
Lactation 135
Lead poisoning 3
Left ventricular
dysfunction 33, 135
ejection fraction 33, 39
hypertrophy 4, 20, 21, 32, 85, 110, 111, 132
Lethargy 136
Liddle's syndrome 3
Lipid profile 75
derangements 43
Lisinopril 33
Liver
disease
acute 136
chronic 136
enzymes, elevated 89
failure 50
function test 75
Lixivaptan 43
Loop diuretics 43-45
Losartan 34
Low-density lipoprotein 32, 138
cholesterol 111
Lower extremity artery disease 5
Lower limb Doppler 21

M

Magnesium 43
sulfate 91
Magnetic resonance
angiography 140
imaging 5, 21, 94
Meditation 27
Mercury sphygmomanometer 5, 6f
Metabolic syndrome 50, 65, 67, 135
Metanephrines 75
Methyldopa 89, 90
Metolazone 43, 44
Metoprolol 49
Microalbuminuria 4, 110
Mineralocorticoid receptor antagonists 35, 86, 133
Minoxidil 53, 55

Mitogen-activated protein kinase 66
Monoamine oxidase inhibitors 3, 78
Moxonidine 53
Multidrug therapy 57
Murmurs 20
Myocardial hypertrophy 32
Myocardial infarction 1, 19, 21, 32, 39, 85, 109, 110, 113
Myocyte hypertrophy 32

N

Nadolol 48
Nausea 43
Nebivolol 49
Nephron 42f
Nervous system 20
Neurofibromatosis, café-au-lait patches of 20
Neurologic hypertensive emergency 77
Neuropathy 80
Neutropenia 33
New York Heart Association 84
    Classification for Heart Failure 84, 84t
Nicardipine 77, 104
Nifedipine 38, 39, 75, 89-91
Nitinol device 139
Nitric oxide 49, 66, 96
Nitroglycerin 76-78, 104, 105
Nitroprusside 77, 89, 104, 112
Nocturia 19
Nondihydropyridines 38t
Nonhealing wound 19
Nonpharmacological therapy 141
Nonsteroidal anti-inflammatory
    agents 3
    drugs 19, 22, 43

O

Obesity 65, 111
Obstructive airways disease 116, 118t
Obstructive sleep apnea 12, 21
Office blood pressure
    classification of 2t
    screening, frequency for 14t
Olmesartan 34

Oral contraceptive 19, 22
Organ system 88
Ototoxicity 43
Overweight 82
Oxidative stress 32

P

Palpitations 19
Parathyroid
    disorders 21
    hormone 22
Parenchymal diseases 3
Perindopril 33
Perindoprilat 33
Perioperative hypertension 101
    etiology of 102
Peripheral arterial disease 20, 110
Peripheral vascular disease 1, 4, 50, 80, 135
    severe 50
Pharmacological therapy 131
Pharmacotherapy 131-133
    initiation of 131
Phenoxybenzamine 53
Phentolamine 77
Pheochromocytoma 3, 20, 21, 75, 124
Plasma
    aldosterone concentration 124
    renin activity 124
Plasminogen activator inhibitor 66
Pneumatic sphygmomanometer 7, 7f
Polycystic kidney disease 3, 19, 20
Polyneuritis 3
Polyuria 19
Porphyria 3
Posterior reversible encephalopathy
    syndrome 77, 89
Postmyocardial infarction 34, 49, 135
Postprandial blood sugar 21, 133
Potassium 25, 32, 43, 132
    sparing diuretics 45
Pranayama 27
Prazosin 53, 75, 136
Preeclampsia 88
Pregnancy 34, 88, 90, 90t, 135, 136
Prerenal azotemia 43
Prinzmetal angina 39, 50

Propranolol 48
Prostatic hypertrophy 136
Protein leak 32
Proteinuria 4, 32, 36, 89, 94, 135
Proximal convoluted tubule 42, 43
Pulse pressure 113

R

Radiofrequency 57
Ramipril 33
Ramiprilat 33
Raynaud's phenomenon 39, 50
Red blood cell 104
Renal artery
    dissection 59
    Doppler 75
    stenosis 59
        bilateral 34, 135
Renal cortical necrosis 89
Renal denervation 58b, 60, 61
    symplicity catheter system for 59f
    therapy 57
        landmark trials of 60, 60t
Renal failure 33, 34, 50
Renal function
    impaired 5
    test 75, 123
Renal nerve denervation 125
Renal sympathetic denervation therapy 139
Renal sympathetic nervous system 58f
    anatomy of 57
    physiology of 57
Renal ultrasound 5
Renin-angiotensin aldosterone system 31, 66, 81, 82, 90, 94
    blockers 112
Reserpine 53
Retinal therapies 19
Retinopathy 80
    hypertensive 4, 5
Rostral ventrolateral medulla 58

S

Salt reduction 130
S-amlodipine 39

Satavaptan 43
Secondary hypertension 2, 3, 20, 21, 21t
    causes of 3
    etiology of 3t
Seizures 89
Sepsis 80
Serum sodium 132
Shavasana 27
Shirshasana 27
Shock, cardiogenic 50
Sinoatrial node 39
Skeletal muscles 66
Skin
    necrosis 50
    rashes 33
Sodium 32, 43
    nitroprusside 76, 77, 105
    potassium adenosine triphosphatase 97
    pump 97
Solitary tract, nucleus of 58
Sotalol 48
Spinal cord section, acute 3
Spironolactone 43, 44, 86, 90
Spontaneous aneurysmal subarachnoid hemorrhage 71
Stenosis 4
Stroke 1, 19, 32, 80
    hemorrhagic 4, 5
    ischemic 4, 5, 70
Subcapsular bleeding 89
Subclinical hypertension-mediated organ damage 110
Sublingual nifedipine 71
Super oxide dismutase 96, 99
Sympatholytics, central 53-55
Syncope 19
Systematic coronary risk evaluation system 110, 110t

T

Tachyarrhythmia 135
Tachycardia 142
Tachyphylaxis 106
Takayasu's disease 20
Target organ damage 74t
Taste disturbance 33

Telmisartan 34
Terazosin 53
Thiazides 43-45, 90, 121
Thrombosis 32
Thyroid 21
    disease, features of 20
    function test 75
    stimulating hormone 22
Thyroxine 22
Timolol 48
Tolvaptan 43, 44
Torsemide 43, 44
Trandolapril 33
Trandolaprilat 33
Transforming growth factor-beta 97
Transient ischemic attack 4, 5, 19, 71, 80, 110, 137
Triamterene 43, 44
Tricyclic antidepressants 3
Triiodothyronine 22
Tumors
    necrosis factor alpha 66
    renal 3, 20

U

Ultrasonography 21, 22, 94
Urinary tract infection 19, 59
Urinary vanillylmandelic acid 75

Urine
    albumin 5
    examination 75

V

Valsartan 34
Vascular disease 4, 5
Vasoconstriction 32
Vasodilators 53, 55, 136
Vasovagal reaction 59
Verapamil 38, 39, 89
Vertigo 19
Vision, blurring of 19
Visual hallucinations 50

W

Water retention 32
Weight 26
    gain 50
    loss 82
    reduction 130
White-coat hypertension 12f, 12t, 122
World Health Organization 65, 129

Y

Yoga 27

EU GSPR Authorised Reprsentative
Logos Europe, 9 rue Nicolas Poussin
1700, La Rochelle, France
Phone: +33 (0) 6 67 93 73 78
E-mail: contact@logoseurope.eu

www.ingramcontent.com/pod-product-compliance
Ingram Content Group UK Ltd.
Pitfield, Milton Keynes, MK11 3LW, UK
UKHW050455150426
5217IPUK00025B/1691